THE ART OF LISTENING

The Art of Listening

By Dominick A. Barbara, M.D., F.A.P.A.

There is an art of listening. To be able really to listen, one should abandon or put aside all prejudices, pre-formulations and daily activities. When you are in a receptive state of mind, things can be easily understood; you are listening when your real attention is given to something. But unfortunately most of us listen through a screen of resistance. We are screened with prejudices, whether religious or spiritual, psychological or scientific; or with our daily worries, desires and fears. And with these for a screen, we listen. Therefore, we listen really to our own noise, to our own sound, not to what is being said. It is extremely difficult to put aside our training, our prejudices, our inclination, our resistance, and, reaching beyond the verbal expression, to listen so that we understand instantaneously. That is going to be one of our difficulties.

—J. Krishnamurti: *The First and Last Personal Freedom*—Harper & Co.

THE ART OF LISTENING

Fourth Printing

By

DOMINICK A. BARBARA, M.D., F.A.P.A.

Certified Practicing Psychoanalyst
Associated with the American Institute for Psychoanalysis
Fellow, American Psychiatric Association
Member, Medical Board of Karen Horney Clinic
Speech Consultant, Long Island Consultation Center
President, American Psychological Speech and Hearing Association

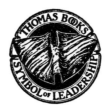

CHARLES C THOMAS • PUBLISHER
Springfield • Illinois • U.S.A.

Published and Distributed Throughout the World by

CHARLES C THOMAS • PUBLISHER

Bannerstone House

301-327 East Lawrence Avenue, Springfield, Illinois, U.S.A.

© *1958, by* CHARLES C THOMAS • PUBLISHER

ISBN 0-398-00086-7

Library of Congress Catalog Card Number: 58-14063

First Printing, 1958
Second Printing, 1966
Third Printing, 1971
Fourth Printing, 1974

With THOMAS BOOKS careful attention is given to all details of manufacturing and design. It is the Publisher's desire to present books that are satisfactory as to their physical qualities and artistic possibilities and appropriate for their particular use. THOMAS BOOKS will be true to those laws of quality that assure a good name and good will.

Printed in the United States of America

R-1

*Dedicated to the memory
of my mother*

Contents

The Art of Listening 1

Listening with the Outer Ear 14

Listening with the Inner Ear (Listening to Ourselves). . 32

Listening with a Receptive Ear (Listening to Others) . . 49

The Magic of Listening 65

Listening to the Essence of Things 80

The Disease of Not Listening 97

Listening with a Modest Ear 113

Listening with a Rebellious Ear 126

Listening with a Deaf Ear 138

Listening with the Third Ear 151

The Sound of Silence 166

When We Stop Listening 182

THE ART OF LISTENING

The Art of Listening

In listening mood she seemed to stand,
The guardian naiad of the strand—

SIR WALTER SCOTT

LISTENING is an art. To be well performed, it requires more than just letting sound waves enter passively into the ear. Good listening is an alive process demanding alert and active participation.

As an art then, it requires knowledge and effort. It is in essence a mental skill which is developed primarily through training and practice. If we are to learn to know how to listen well, we must proceed as we would in learning any other art such as music, painting, architecture or acting. We must inquire about all the basic essentials of productive listening; and that done, we must practice faithfully until we have mastered the techniques.

The art of listening is not something we can acquire through "do-it-yourself" shortcuts. The good listener "listens between the lines. He constantly applies his spare thinking to what is being said."[1] And while he is attentive to what is being said, he is also aware of the total facts at hand, both in their verbal connotations and their nonverbal implications.

First of all, the practice of an art requires *discipline*. It is essential, writes Fromm, "that discipline should not be practiced like a rule imposed on oneself from the outside, but that it becomes an expression of one's own will; that it is felt as pleasant, and that one slowly accustoms one-

1

self to a kind of behavior which one would eventually miss, if one stopped practicing it."[2] It is imperative that we be in the mood to want to listen and at the same time consider some of its more challenging aspects. It would be well were we to devote a period of each day to serious listening, this in contrast to the vast amount of superficial listening we indulge in when we meet in various social groups or during frequent coffee breaks.

Concentration is a second prerequisite of good listening. Most of us have difficulty in concentrating. We take a peculiar pride in doing a number of things at the same time. We watch television *and* read *and* talk *and* smoke *and* eat *and* drink. Lack of concentration is also prevalent because of our fear of being alone with ourselves. We find it well nigh impossible to sit still, to be silent, to concentrate on something specific for any length of time. We become nervous and fidgety and to allay our anxieties, we turn to almost any form of hectic or compulsive activity.

In order to concentrate fully when listening, we should be *patient* with ourselves. This virtue is as difficult to cultivate as discipline and concentration. In an age of speed reinforced by the use of the airplane, telephone, radio and television, modern man is trained to think that he loses out on time when he pauses to concentrate. He feels compelled to listen only to those facts he digests quickly and is able to keep at his finger tips with as little effort or concentration as possible. To linger on in reflection over a certain situation or fact goes against his idealized concept of himself as "a man of action."

In learning to concentrate, it is most important that we remove distractions in the path of our listening. We can then be alone with our innermost feelings and thoughts and can give to ourselves and our surroundings our whole interest and attention. By concentrating intensely we can keep our ears fully opened to all aural stimuli, and at the same time be curious and alert enough to tune in to

2

our proper wave lengths. We can then listen without too much confusion, apprehension or mental interference.

In listening, it is essential that we give our full attention to the situation at hand. By so doing, we learn to live fully in the present, in the *here* and *now* and to evaluate things as they *are*. This will also mean less indulgence in trivial talk and more time for the serious exchange of ideas, feelings and opinions. In this way, we shall become increasingly sensitive to ourselves and to other people's wishes, thoughts and beliefs.

Good listening demands active participation. It involves keeping one's mind in a state of relaxed alertness, open and flexible to all relevant changes in a given situation. To listen with an active and open mind also entails giving a speaker a chance to present all the facts involved rather than allowing ourselves to jump to premature conclusions. The effectual listener is constantly on the alert to find something interesting in what is being said and attempts to keep the discussion moving and alive either by asking productive questions or by adding something constructive to the situation as a whole. The ineffectual listener, on the other hand, is on the defensive, planning rebuttals or questions designed to embarrass or belittle the speaker, or using his attack to further only his own selfish motives.

The productive listener develops his listening skill to the degree that he can direct his full attention to the basic idea. He learns to utilize this ability constructively by focusing his energies toward the true meaning or theme of a situation instead of getting lost by seeking to remember every fact as it is presented. He is also less impressed by the persuasive power of the spoken word or the superficialities of the speaker, and is more concerned with getting to the heart of the matter.

A third factor contributing to the effectiveness of listening is that of *comprehension*, the understanding and grasp of the true idea or meaning of what is heard. When the facts one hears and the principles that are deduced from what is being said or implied lead in turn to levels of agreement between the listener and the speaker on whatever is being discussed, then effective listening has been achieved.

Comprehension in any given situation is to be found not in the words that are spoken, but in the meaning given by both the sender and the receiver. If properly attuned to each other, both will break through the barrier of intellectualization and arrive at true meaning and understanding. Both will leave the situation feeling satisfied and wiser.

Comprehension in listening is difficult because we think faster than we talk. As has been reported, the rate of speech of most Americans is about 125 words a minute. Yet we think four times that fast. This discrepancy leaves a lot of time for spare thinking. It is what we do with this extra time that makes us either good or poor listeners. If we are poor listeners, to quote Nichols and Stevens, "we soon become impatient; our thoughts turn to something else for a moment, then dart back to the speaker. These brief side excursions continue until our mind tarries too long on some other subject. Then, when our thoughts return to the person talking, we find he's far ahead of us. Now it's harder to follow him and increasingly easy to take off on our side excursions. Finally we give up; the person is still talking, but our mind is in another world."[3]

The good listener in contrast is selective and uses his spare thinking time to advantage by asking himself what is being said, in what context is it being said, and how accurate the speaker's facts are. He also tries to be as much alone with his thoughts and feelings as possible so that he can concentrate and listen with little prejudice, condemnation or criticism. He makes a genuine effort to reach beyond the actual words that are spoken and get at the basic meaning by visualizing the situation as a whole. To comprehend fully then, it is essential that one sharpen his listening skill to the point where he is interested in what he is listening to and, at the same time, avoid being easily distracted.

Comprehension may be loosely defined as the ability to recall immediately or at some later time a sampling of what has been read or heard. Rarely does it take into account what the individual does with the retained material, nor does it emphasize the critical and creative evaluation of what is received. In our schools and colleges, for instance, such a definition of comprehension according to Johnson, "does not encourage one to develop the implications of the message nor to extend and refine it. It encourages the student to listen the way a tape recorder 'listens'—and consequently to speak the way a tape recorder 'speaks.' It is as though the instructor were to talk 'into his students' on Monday and Wednesdays and to 'play them back' in a quiz on Friday." [4]

As human beings we may desire to hear only what we want to hear and to discard anything else we do not want to hear. This interferes with good listening. To remedy this situation, we must try to see less of the world from within ourselves and be more objective. This can be accomplished by improving our faculty to see people and things *as they actually are*. We can thus separate this objective picture from just any picture which may have been formed by our own inner illusions, anxieties and fears.

To acquire this capacity for objectivity when listening, we must "hear the other person out" without imposing our preconceived notions or opinions. This requires reason, humility and a degree of self-control. Since the objective is to comprehend most of what the speaker is saying, we must learn to hold back our own judgments and decisions until after he has finished. Only then can we honestly reach a true evaluation of what was said. Having listened to our fullest capacity, we can now summarize, digest and

5

evaluate within ourselves what is of importance to us and to the situation as a whole. A realistic self-evaluation achieved, agreement occurs between speaker and listener and true communication takes place.

To listen and to think actively one must have an alert mind and plenty of native curiosity sustained by many interests. Inner vitality is an emotional source or fuel which enables the thinking mind to develop. A person living in a stimulating atmosphere of intellectual interests will seek more and more information to foster his further growth. He will develop the habit of concentrating and actively applying his listening skill to its fullest capacity. He will listen more and better, in order to more effectively comprehend and understand the world about him. As he does so, he reaches out toward a clearer and deeper experiencing of himself.

Communicative Aspects of Good Listening

In a recent article, "The Integrity of the Listener," Richard Henry considers successful communication as a function not only of agreement on the meaning of words or phrases, but also of consideration of the fact that there are patterns of thought and meaning that condition one's reactions to the statements of others. Effective communication comes therefore from the comprehension that the same words often mean different things to different people, depending upon their experience and their patterns of thought and conceptions. Words in themselves have little or no intrinsic meaning. Their meaning is largely determined by the context in which they appear, and that context "is at least a two-dimensional one: the context of the speaker, and the context of the listener,—each of them slightly different." [5]

When listening we have to consider the nuances of meaning of different languages, the specific context within which words are used to convey meaning, and the emotional tone of the speaker and the attitudes this tone conveys. For instance, when disagreement occurs and communication breaks down between two people, it is important to look not just at the disagreement itself but also at the mood in which it is expressed. If you offer a point of view or an assertion to someone and his expressed disagreement conveys back to you the impression that he considers you ignorant or misled, communication has failed. In other words, in listening with arrogance or prejudice, we distort the true intent of the message by misleading our speaker with our self-imposed attitudes.

To listen effectively, verbal affirmation of our feelings or attitudes is not enough. For understanding to result, there must be sincere effort expended on the part of the listener. He must be patient, open-minded and, to some degree, enter genuinely into the emotional life of the speaker.

For communication to be effective, its network must be functionally organized and the flow of messages be adapted to the capacity of both the speaker and the listener. Information which flows from one person to another is said to have content only when sender and receiver can reach levels of agreement regarding the statement or subject matter at hand. It further entails the use of this information for knowledge which enables those involved to reconstruct past events, predict future events, and so engage in successful action.

Correct evaluations of the past and appropriate decisions for the future are largely based upon the relevance, accuracy and completeness of such information. In this particular aspect of communication, listening plays a most important role. To evaluate efficiently what someone else is attempting to convey, we must take into account not only what we hear from the outside, but whatever additional information comes to us simultaneously from our inner wishes, feelings and beliefs. It is in the appropriate handling of both this outside perspective and the messages from our inner sources that we can effectively arrive at a correct evaluation of whatever information we have obtained.

The efficiency of a communication system depends to a large extent upon the feedback circuits and the use to which they are put. For example, in listening to a particular speaker, if the effect of his message upon us is so received that it provokes disagreement or little response at all, then something is defective in the communication system. For people to relate to each other, it is essential that they favorably influence each other. When we cease to listen effectively or do not relay favorable influences back to others, our relationships are disturbed. We stop learning; we do not bring our information up to date and so feed back faulty messages to others. Such disturbances in the feedback mechanism tend to cause a gradual breakdown in the communication system.

Successful communication also depends upon the co-operation of at least two or more people. In this context, the listener also plays a specific role. His attitude, when listening effectively, is one of curiosity and eagerness to find out what the effects of a statement or an action might have been. He makes efforts at the same time to consider other individuals and groups in terms of whether or not they will be able to cope with the effects of a projected statement or an anticipated action. A good listener works incessantly toward facilitating and improving the feedback mechanism. He attempts to visualize situations as a whole and he keeps alive the communicative process by asking others for suggestions and incorporating these in his future actions.

A listener, sincere in his desire to facilitate the efficiency of communication with others, is highly selective and times his responses so that his receivers are capable of perceiving and interpreting them without undue difficulty or haste.

He is alert to necessary corrections in the information from others or to the need from within himself for clarity, distinctness and relevance. He is less interested in the "why" or "what" of a message than he is in the "how" of communication. This leads to better discussion and understanding and thus to healthier relationships.

In listening with purpose, responsibility must be shared by both the speaker and the listener. Both have the same problem in keeping the communicative process alive. Each must also enlighten his own self-interest to the degree that he can facilitate communication with others by making good use of circuit response. In this way the listener's reactions help the speaker and make it easier for him to bring out what he wishes to convey and, in the last analysis, to improve total communication.

In effective communication, the language used must be clear, concise, simple and flexible in nature. In relating to others, we express our opinions, feelings, beliefs or awareness to the degree to which our thoughts or statements are projective representations of our inner state at the particular time of expression. For a language therefore to be meaningful, it must in itself be variable, flexible, and in dynamic change from person to person and situation to situation, and at the same time have clarity for both speaker and listener.

In order to become better listeners and to give our lives a constructive and purposeful meaning, it is essential that we talk simply and understand clearly. Since speech is the essential means of communication, mutual understanding must depend upon *shared* meanings. Meaning is relative to experience and in order that a message be understood there must be an overlapping of experience between sender and receiver. Also, the cultivation of a productive language will enable us to listen to and understand the implied meanings behind words, names and labels. As we gain a better knowledge of the structure

9

of the world we live in, its complexities will grow less mysterious and confused; and in time, as we communicate with each other in truthful meaning, a sense of responsibility, mutual rapport and understanding will develop and grow.

The Listener as an Individual

Man is a communicating animal. Much of what he achieves in his understanding of others depends upon the degree to which he is able to verbalize his thoughts, wishes and feelings. On the other hand, real communication or relatedness between people becomes difficult if there is present a lack of desire for genuine communion or concern for others as individuals. Henry says the aim of real communication "is a kind of communion with the other person, a sharing of one's self and an appreciation for the other which affirms the integrity of each. Real understanding comes, we might say, where there's an unspoken agreement that each recognizes the right to self-hood of the other, a self-hood which is unique, and accepted and rejoiced in as such,—and further, which eagerly desires the other more fully and deeply than he does before the process of communication begins."[6]

The mere acceptance of others is but the beginning of communication. There must be a full acceptance of the other person, a communion with him as *he is*, a relinquishing of any preconceived image of this same person that may have been created in the mind of another. We are creatures of habit, so subjected to past experience and to pulls from emotional forces within ourselves that we see or hear only what we want to and then in terms of our individual beliefs, thoughts or desires. We tend to create these images of others from the things they say or do over the period of our acquaintance with them, and from what we know of their social standing, jobs, religion or family backgrounds.

With long acquaintance, we tend to arrive at the point of predicting and anticipating the other person's reactions to such and such a problem or situation and to make guesses about what he will think or do or say under certain conditions. We systematize our thinking and listening to the point that we make ourselves believe that we cannot expect this or that person to react in any way but the way he's behaved in the past under similar conditions. We create images in our own imaginations of people as we *think* they are and in so doing we are often gravely in error in terms of reality.

Communication becomes more effective as we see and listen to others as they appear realistically. It is essential that we see others as unique personalities, with beliefs, thoughts and wishes of their own, whose capacities for thinking and experiencing are constantly changing, growing, developing into something new and stimulating. Genuine understanding is dependent, above all else, on this *eagerness to affirm the integrity of others.*

In productive listening, it is essential that we not place screens or facades in the way of our arriving at the truth of the matter. In *The Brothers Karamazov*, Dostoyevsky wrote: ". . . The man who lies to himself and listens to his own lies comes to such a pass that he cannot distinguish the truth within him, or around him, and so loses all respect for himself and for others . . . ."

When listening to others, we must strive toward mutual communication and mutual understanding. In a real conversation we are not conscious of who is talking, who is listening. We are lost in the total communicative atmosphere. As we relax, come closest to our feelings, and arrive at free verbal intercourse, productivity reaches its highest peak; our listening becomes highly selective, and we become more aware and attuned to the essence of the facts or situation at hand. We reach mutual levels of agreement where we favorably influence each other.

We learn from such a communication situation and so leave it both wiser and healthier.

Inherent in man, according to Horney, "are evolutionary constructive forces, which urge him to realize his given potentialities . . . It means that man, by his very nature and of his own accord, strives toward self-realization, and that his set of values evolves from such striving. Apparently he cannot, for example, develop his full human potentialities unless he is truthful to himself; unless he is active and productive; unless he relates to himself and to others in the spirit of mutuality."[7]

In listening with meaning, we must constantly seek to gain an ever increasing awareness and understanding of ourselves and others. In this sense, self-knowledge becomes not an aim in itself but a means of liberating the forces of spontaneous growth. To grow we must assume responsibility for ourselves. We can, in this sense, accept working at ourselves as a *moral privilege* rather than as a prime moral *obligation*. The more we take our growth seriously, the more we will develop the desire to do so. And the more we get rid of our own neurotic shackles, the freer we will become to grow within ourselves, and to love and have concern for others. Thus we shall acquire a rational faith which will have the certainty and firmness of our own convictions, and this will pervade our entire concept of life.

For listening to be effective as an art, we must be active participants in its whole process. This means not only working just through our ears. It also means responding holistically with our full hearing capacity and our inner perceptions. It entails being fully attentive and awake, alert at every minute to screen out inner prejudices, condemnations or preconceived notions. It means being active in thought and feeling and with one's eyes and ears to avoid inertia. It means being open and receptive to others. It demands of us an enhanced vitality, an aliveness, and a firm desire to commune with others. With all this in hand, we shall grow healthily as human beings, able to influence others with meaning. So we shall arrive at a sustained level of mutual and truthful communication.

References

1. Ralph G. Nichols and Leonard A. Stevens: *Are You Listening?* New York, McGraw-Hill Book Company, 1957, p. 83.
2. Erich Fromm: *The Art of Loving.* New York, Harper & Bros., 1956, p. 111.
3. Ralph B. Nichols and Leonard A. Stevens: *op. cit.*, p. 151.
4. Wendell Johnson: *Your Most Enchanted Listener.* New York, Harper & Bros., 1956, p. 195.
5, 6. Richard Henry: "The Integrity of the Listener," *Today's Speech*, Sept. 1957, Vol. 5, No. 3.
7. Karen Horney: *Neurosis & Human Growth.* New York, Norton & Company, 1950, p. 15.

Listening with the Outer Ear

He that hath ears to hear,
Let him hear.

—MARK IV

IN his stimulating book, *Conversation and Communication*, Meerloo says, "Our sound world is related to the world of rhythm and time. It brings us the awareness of history and continuity . . . . The visual picture is imbued with reality. Hearing, however, acts more deeply than seeing. Seeing is virtually touching; it is always initiated by material reality and concrete situations. Hearing involves a much finer selection of spiritual values; we can never come back to it. The spoken sound disappears. We cannot verify it again and again."[1]

The symbolic meaning of the ear has been elaborated on in myth and literature. In early Christian writings and in medieval art, for instance, the Conception of Jesus was often depicted as being caused by the entrance of the Holy Spirit, usually in the guise of a bird, into Mary's ear. This legendary function of the ear has been further recorded in early paintings and in epic poetry wherein both the Devil and the sea serpent ingested their victims through the mouth and eliminated them through the cloaca or the ear or both. Such illustrations, according to Ernest Jones, show the receptive ear serves as a displacement for the foul anal region, thereby making the carnal act clean and pure. He then compares this ancient concept to our own use of the ear as a receiver of "clean wind, intangible sound and the abstract word."

14

The ear, however, is more than just a receptive opening. Symbolically we connote to it meaningful representations of strength, curiosity or sex. For example, we speak of "listening with our good ear" when we are interested in hearing something of value to us; we refer to "pricking up our ears" when we are attentive or curious; children "wiggle" their ears; ears are "boxed" by irate parents; and in the vernacular, they are "pinned back" to denote defeat. In this same context, it was said, Midas, King of Phrygia, was given an ass's ears by Apollo for preferring, in a contest, the music of Marsyas to the gods'. Midas preserved his shame from all but his barber who, wishing to tell it, whispered into a hole in the ground. In time the reeds which grew out of that hole repeated the words and so exposed the secret to the world. It is said that Midas was punished not for his earlier greed but for abuse of his ears which, in hearing too avidly the sounds of Pan, had failed to listen to the authority of the gods.

For centuries the ear has been a vital area of sexual significance. From prehistoric times the earring has been considered as a personal adornment. Among earring forms used are the ball, crescent, chain, plaque, sacred symbols and representations of animals—the size and length changing with the fashion. The Egyptians favored a gold hoop-earring and, later, the incrusted pendant. In Babylonia and Assyria the earring evolved into an exquisite work of the goldsmith's art and was developed with great richness in Persia, India and the Far East. In the East it has been worn by men to denote rank.

Even now some primitive tribes distort the ear lobe with plugs several inches in diameter or with heavy stones. The Masai still use ear plugs four and a half inches in diameter, weighing almost three pounds in order to stretch their ears. The ruling class of the Inca called *orejones* or "Big Ears" by the Spaniards pierced their ears and enlarged the holes until the lobes hung almost to their shoulders. To this day, Hopi girls wear small turquoise earrings with a peculiar arrangement of the hair which symbolizes the squash blossom, while the men wear gigantic earrings supposedly representing their genital formation.

Man is primarily a talking animal. The more complex and differentiated he has become, the more essential is his need for a specialized system of communication. Among the lower animals, insects and birds, communication is primarily on a sensory or extrasensory basis. Bats, for instance, make use of supersonic sounds and echo effects. Bees utilize refined smell and dancing actions in order to communicate direction. Von Frisch has found through a series of careful experiments that bees returning to a hive inform their fellows of the distance and direction of a feeding place by wagging dances on the vertical comb, the direction being indicated by the angle at which they point in their dance.

Man, like the dog, was essentially at one time a "smell" animal. However through the centuries man, like the ape, has gradually become an "eye" animal. Man primarily *looks* instead of *sniffing* around. But whereas the dog's hearing has so improved with time that, with his delicately attuned ears, he can listen to sounds much too refined for the human ear, man has not learned to utilize his hearing to the fullest capacity. Consequently his ears have not yet been trained to take in the finer nuances of sound. As a result, it is only in the past few years that listening has begun to assume greater importance among us.

Listening is an art which has been highly neglected. We all are compelled in one way or another today to maintain verbalized activity as reflected in the constant flow of chatter and gossip of communal life. The Zulus, for example, still use the so-called "filling sounds" in order to keep their mouths busy. In their long sentences only a few words have specific meaning; the rest are used to fill in the voids. In children we find this same effect reached in the babbling and prattling which in essence is not communication but simply playing with noises. There are some organized "palavers" in primitive tribes, meetings in which prolonged indulgence in words and debate occurs, often without any decision being reached. Not even the threat of famine will disrupt this verbal spree which fosters a kind of ecstatic anaesthesia. It requires the magic ceremonial of the witch doctors to initiate more useful and necessary activities such as hunting and fishing; and once such activities have been completed, the tribe invariably returns to a chattering inactivity. As Meerloo puts it, "the music of words brings them oblivion."[2]

The Human Ear

A most marvelous and complex organ of the human body is the ear. How many of you have ever wondered how one hears? Just lift up your head and listen. When a Stradivarius is well played, the sound waves pass from the violin through the air to the ear. From here on in, providing you are free of ear troubles, these sound waves are converted into electrical impulses in the auditory nerve and then relayed along the entire complicated hearing apparatus. What usually results is that we hear a beautiful blend of sounds, more delicate than any modern hi-fi can ever hope to reproduce, this because the ear has an amazing acoustic sensitivity, much finer than any instrument can approximate.

The organ of hearing consists of three parts: the outer visible ear, the middle ear with its eardrum, and the inner ear. The *inner ear* is the true sense-organ. It is here that the vibrations cause the excitation of sensory cells and the initiation of the nervous impulses, whereas the outer and middle ears are structures which, in collecting and transmitting sound vibrations to the inner ear, make it possible

17

for this complicated and delicate device to lie safely embedded in the bone of the skull. Most mammals are equipped with a natural ear-trumpet in the external ear. This is a hollow cone which can readily be turned about to face the direction from which sounds are coming, thereby making feeble sounds more distinctly audible. From this ear-trumpet a short tube leads to the eardrum or boundary separating the outer and middle ears. In man, this amplifying apparatus is poorly developed and the external ear is little more than a mere flap of no acoustic importance. The power to move or regulate it with but few exceptions is absent. Thus, although a person may distinguish sounds varying over a wide range of pitch, he is less able to discern faint sounds than a dog or a horse, and he therefore has no accurate idea of the direction from which the sounds are coming. The tube from the external ear to the eardrum is also provided with hairs and wax-secreting cells that have a filtering and protecting function similar to that of the hairs and mucus-secreting cells of the nose.

The *middle ear* is a narrow chamber filled with air and communicating with the mouth by means of a duct, known as the *Eustachian tube.* This tube is constructed in such a way that it functions like a one-way valve. Its walls are usually pressed flat together, but when the pressure in the middle ear varies too greatly from that outside, they are forced open and a little air passes one way or the other. Almost everyone has experienced the slight fullness in the ears which occurs with a change in altitude as in a fast-rising elevator or on an auto trip over mountains. These sensations are ordinarily of no importance, signifying only changes in the pressure of the air in the middle ear.

The walls of the middle ear are strong and bony except in three places. The first and largest of these is the eardrum. In the second and third, the *fenestra ovalis* and

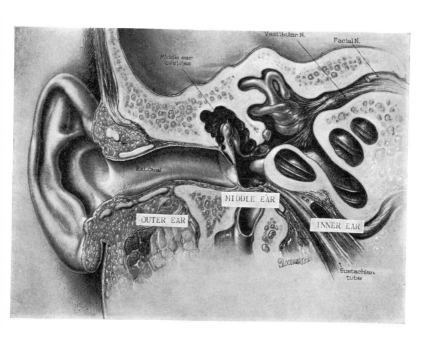

fenestra rotunda (oval window and round window), there are even more delicate membranes which separate the middle and inner ears. A series of three small bones which occupy the cavity of the middle ear, called the ear ossicles, are the *malleus* (hammer), the *incus* (anvil) and the *stapes* (stirrup). This last bone of the chain has its internal base in flexible contact with the fluid of the inner ear. The motion transmitted to this fluid in turn stimulates the nerve endings situated in the actual organ of hearing, the *cochlea*. Nerve currents are set up which are then carried by the auditory nerve to the brain.

Actually sound waves travel a rather circuitous route through the ear. Hearing begins with auditory stimuli passing through the air to the ear. The sound waves pass into the ear and make the eardrum, which is stretched tight like a drum skin, vibrate. This in turn transmits vibrations to the *fenestra ovalis*. This latter elaborate device is partly protective, for the *malleus* is so jointed to the *incus* that if a violent jar such as a box on the ear occurs, the two are disengaged and the shock is blocked from passing on to the more delicate inner structures. The inner ear is filled with a water fluid. The properties of sound waves moving in water are very different from those travelling in air. Now the ear bones act primarily as levers and reduce the amplitude of the vibrations, yet by at the same time concentrating the energy of the vibrating eardrum onto a window only one-twentieth its size, the sound waves become more vigorous. This is one way in which the human ear attempts to cope with the problem of transmitting sound waves from air to water.

The *inner ear* is an elaborate labyrinth of passages embedded in bone and filled with a lymph-like fluid. The only part of the inner ear concerned with hearing is a narrow, tapering tube about an inch long which is coiled into a dwindling spiral like the shell of a snail. Appropriately called the *cochlea*, this is divided into three compartments by a partition which runs along its whole length.

On this partition are situated the sensitive endings of the ear nerves. These sense cells are made up of stiff hair-like projections which are surrounded by the endings of nerve fibres. They are placed anatomically on an elastic membrane and overhung by a rigid shelf. When the fluid surrounding the apparatus vibrates, the elastic membrane bounces up and down and the sense cells are brought into collision with the rigid shelf. It is this impact with the shelf that stimulates the cells and causes them to relay impulses along the nerve fibres to the brain.

According to the authors of a most informative book, *The Science of Life*,[3] the following is the theory most extensively held regarding the method of discriminating between sounds of different pitch. The diameter of the cochlea decreases steadily from end to end of the spiral much as a spiral staircase dwindles to a point at the top. Since all the structures inside must necessarily decrease in proportion, the width of the elastic membrane on which the sense cells are placed also decreases. Thus, since the period of vibration of an elastic body varies with its size, the different parts of this membrane are tuned to different notes. The apparatus in essence is like a piano or harp whose wires produce notes of higher pitch as they decrease in length. For instance, it is known that if a tuning fork is sounded near a piano when the damping pedal is down, the particular note of the tuning fork is echoed by the appropriate wire of the piano. In other words, the pulsations emitted by the tuning fork will make a wire vibrate if the wire is tuned to the same pitch.

Just so do rhythmical vibrations of the fluid in the inner ear vibrate only that particular part of the elastic membrane tuned to their own pitch. Thus we see that notes of different pitch may affect different parts of the membrane and so cause impulses to be sent to the brain along different nerve fibres. In the final analysis, it is in the brain that the sensations given by simultaneous notes of different pitch are combined to form the complex sensation of a chord.

As sound waves travel along the complicated route through the ear, there are many factors which may disturb their natural course. Any interference along this route may interfere with normal hearing. An obstruction such as wax in the ear canal changes the vibratory properties of the eardrum. Incorrect pressure in the middle ear caused by a cold, fluid or pus in the middle ear, stiffness of the joints between the ossicles as in otosclerosis, etc., all may impair hearing. Also in rare cases, the nerve endings may be unable to respond to a sound wave because of disease of the main nerve or of the brain's temporal lobe.

The Problem of Impaired Hearing

In an era like the present where "being heard and understood" is so crucial, the number of those who have difficulties in hearing is almost beyond belief. In testing the hearing ability of college students over a number of years, audiologists have found that about four or five out of every hundred have sufficient hearing loss to warrant examination by an ear specialist. Statistically about one out of every hundred persons has a substantial loss of hearing. Furthermore with increasing years, hearing commonly becomes impaired.

Our best estimate from available data (Silverman, 1947) is that five per cent of school-age children have a hearing impairment of some kind, with one or two out of every ten in this group in need of special educational attention. The rest will either respond to medical care or their hearing loss is not apt to reach the handicapping stage. There are, in addition, about 22,100 children in schools for the deaf in the United States, these ranging from the hard of hearing and aphasiacs to those completely deaf.

In spite of the enormity of this problem, Western man's

serious attempts to work with it have been slow and faltering. In the sixth century, the Justinian Code classified the deaf and dumb as mentally incompetent. In the second century B.C. the Rabbis of the Talmud had classified the deaf with fools and children. In the sixteenth century Cardano of Padua was one of the first to assert that the deaf could be taught to comprehend written symbols or combinations of symbols by associating these with the object or picture of the object they were intended to represent. In 1680 Dalgaino introduced the possibility of pre-school education, and de L'Epee of France and Heinicke of Germany argued the merits of the intellectual development of the deaf. Edward Miner Gallaudet brought the French system, a language of signs, to the United States, and in the nineteenth century Alexander Graham Bell applied a science of speech to teaching the deaf. But it is only in recent years that the universality of education opportunity for deaf children of school age has become a reality in our country and today the deaf are progressively becoming economically and socially productive men and women.

Psychological Aspects of Hearing

At birth the child perceives the external world primarily through the intervention of his mechanical and chemical end organs. In the next few years he learns to rely more upon the vision and hearing which enable him to perceive and explore the more distant environment. An inability to make effective use of sensory modality for exploration of this environment, according to Ruesch, is one of the foundations of disturbed communication.

The ears are essentially receptive organs, and therefore the ability to respond to sound is present at birth. The Moro reflex, used to test the integrity of the neonate's reflexes, depends on the capacity to perceive sound waves. The response to a sudden sharp sound or to loss of equilibrium is the only protective reaction associated with a special sense that is present at birth. The sense of hearing, like that of seeing, is closely related to the infant's ability to identify or to separate himself from his environment. Though present earlier in embryonic development, it is a less acute perceptor than that of sight.

The infant uses his hearing to distinguish sounds which come from himself or those which originate from some outside source. The gurgling or cooing which acts as a primary form of communication between mother and infant is part of the total communication in which sound plays an important role. However, apart from its unifying action, the loss of the function of hearing has a separating effect on the individual. When the sense of hearing is impaired or completely gone, the victim's personality feels estranged from the outside environment. In the more severe cases of deafness, this can lead to psychosis.

Emotionally the ear is also the organ through which the verbal taboos and restrictions of the parents are communicated to the child. Words like "bad," "dirty," "naughty," etc. used to discipline the child through the intonation and the intensity of their utterance, are all transmitted to the child's psyche through the ear. A common response of the child to verbal abuse is to clap both hands over his ears to shut out such disciplining sounds made by the parent.

In the child there is early evidence of auditory adaptation. The one week old child is startled by loud noises—he soon blinks at sharp sounds. At about one month, he may be perceptive to voice and music and be quieted by the sound of talking or singing. At four months he turns his head in the direction of voices heard, and at six months, toward a ringing bell. At approximately nine months he begins to adjust to words. His audition is now complete enough to aid the infant in the acquisition of language and in the finer discrimination of sounds.[5]

23

Fears in children develop mainly at the ages when the organism is actively crossing frontiers into strange new territories. Susceptibility also changes in type. There is a trend in emphasis from *auditory* (2-2½ years) to *spatial*, to *visual* (3 years), to *auditory* (4-5½ years), to *personal* (7 years).

Even within any one type of fear, significant developmental changes occur. Let us consider fears of sounds. At first, Gesell and Ilg[10] have found, the child fears loud or sudden sounds or those outside his natural range (1-6 months); then sounds of mechanical gadgets (18 months); sounds of trains, trucks, flushing toilets, barking dogs (2-2½ years); fire engines (4 years); rain and thunder (5 years); doorbell, telephone, static, ugly voices, bird and insect noises (5½-6 years).

An infant fears sinister sounds—the noise of thunder, rain, wind and fire. Also many of the man-made sounds such as sirens, static, the roar of a vacuum cleaner, telephones, the flushing of the toilet, or a parent's angry voice will induce fear until they are localized and identified. The child may symbolically attempt to protect himself by putting his hands over his ears or by hiding behind his mother's back. But not until he is ten or so does he begin to laugh at these "babyish" fears he has outgrown. Even as he matures, he does not banish fear altogether; he merely has learned to diminish and define the fear and its source.

Invariably deeply engrossed in his own activities, the child readily shifts his attention and often gives the impression of not listening. And the usual complaint made by the mother at such times is that the child is deaf. However, under closer observation, we find that he does respond to the signal of a bell, a change in the tone of voive, a whisper, a magic word or a whistle.

A child is notorious for his involuntary refusal to listen when he does not want to. He may have heard what was

24

said, but he does not respond either because he is so interested in his play or because he feels that doing so isn't important to his own welfare. Only when the tone of the parent's voice indicates sternness or that some punishment is imminent does he respond. When he is subjected to a parental environment where listening is a *must* or where he has tried to mold himself into an obedient and attentive listener, then the child may really not hear when he is called. By blotting out the consciousness of his sensory impressions, he can be disobedient and yet relieve himself of any feeling of guilt about his disobediance.

In more severe situations, this may well become a hysterical deafness—that is, the child actually deafens himself to all or certain specific sounds if they have been associated in his mind with former unpleasant experiences. For example, if a child has overheard parental intercourse and has identified unpleasant feelings with the sounds, he may repress the memory and any sounds that remind him of what he has heard. Children will often react to this repression as if they were actually deaf and since they have not heard to their fullest capacity, they will often compensate by developing a greater sensitivity in another sense such as sight or touch.

Ramsdell has described three psychological levels of hearing: a) the *primitive level* at which we are aware there is sound around us, i.e., the noises of the everyday world; b) the *signal* or *warning level* at which we make use of certain types of auditory information, i.e. the ring of the telephone or the whistle of the traffic policeman; c) the *symbolic level* at which we understand language. He attributes the "depression" of the deaf to absence of hearing on the primitive level because it creates a sense of apartness from the world, while not hearing at the warning level may merely cause a feeling of insecurity. Hearing at the symbolic level essentially enables us to communicate experiences, to clarify and to organize our

25

thoughts to achieve high order knowledge and, in the growing child, "to formalize and to bind those social prohibitions and permissions which make up the moral code."[6]

Deaf children, particularly those deaf from birth, usually have impaired *gestalt* discrimination and a reduced ability to draw human figures, the latter undoubtedly caused by an inadequate perceptual contact with the earliest environment and diminished stimulation by their first sensory love objects. Yet the basic contribution, beyond that of primary language, which audition makes to personality development remains obscure. It is known, however, that hearing helps in developing many special skills which are important in everyday functioning. These skills may apply to primitive living conditions, when blindness occurs, or in particular areas of work such as mechanics, medicine, and in music, where—as an example—our words identify hearing with the talent when we say of the virtuoso that he has a "fine ear."

Failure in acoustic perception can cause difficulties of an emotional nature ranging from mild neurosis to severe states of psychotic intervention. Though there is rarely evidence of gross physical damage in deafness, at a deeper level the failure to function in this area often produces a sense of mutilation. "Hard-of-hearing patients," writes Knapp, "may have a special sensitivity, beyond that fostered by cultural inertia, to wearing the badge of invalidism, a hearing aid, inserted in the opening of their faulty party. Along with special personal defensive attitudes, there is usually some sign of the anxiety one would expect from any lesion—concern over sensations around the ear, drainage from it, or noises in it."[7]

He goes on to give a most interesting case history to illustrate his point:

"A man, fifty-four years old, a plumbing salesman, once enuretic, later an inventor of a 'drip-proof' faucet, came to the clinic because of lifetime concern about his ears, which had changed to near panic following instrumentation of his Eustachian tubes two years ago. He traced all his difficulties to an apparent memory from the age of five, of putting three peas into his right ear, and having a doctor attempt to remove them, only to push one through the drum. From then on, although audiograms showed residual hearing, he felt himself to be totally deaf on that side. He hid his defect, even from his domineering wife, never cupped his ear or turned his head toward a speaker, and felt crippled—'like having only one leg.' He prided himself on exceptionally keen hearing in the left ear, though it made him 'guilty,' and he constantly dreaded losing it, too. At the same time there was a persistent feeling, enhanced by frequent colds, that there was something in his bad ear. After a bloody surgical removal of a urethral stone at age forty-six, he developed a swelling in his nose, which culminated, when he was fifty-two, in removal of a bloody nasal polyp. A month later he got some water in his good ear and became terrified when he 'couldn't get it out.' A doctor tried to dilate his Eustachian tube with a bougie. The patient recalled him 'shoving it in,' and could 'feel the crushing and cracking.' He developed transient deafness, and the thought that his 'ears had been plugged, as if someone had put something in them.' During psychotherapy his acute distress subsided. He lost some of his fears of total deafness; at the same time he felt the bone in his nose was 'growing back,' and he continued to ruminate about the mysterious, threatening events going on inside the passages of his head.

"This patient illustrates the persistent fantasy of the ear as a container, which can be penetrated to result in a growth. But also he had the opposite idea, of a keen ear. Anxiety over losing this hung over his lifelong compromise—in which he felt that one ear was damaged, the other intact, one passive and filled up, the other active and grasping."[7]

It appears that blind persons as a rule endure their affliction more easily than the deaf. One seldom finds that the circumstance of blindness culminates in severe mental illness. According to Isakower,[8] the auditory sphere of man is the last step in a phylogenetic development from the static organ of the crustaceans and is of utmost importance for the regulation of our relations with our environment and for the building up of the super-ego.

Freud, in this same context, has shown the importance of auditory perceptions for verbal images and has disclosed that they are in essence one of the most important requisites for memory-residues and thinking. He has further stated that in infancy our first relationship consists only of a primary identification with outside objects, and that to a certain extent in all later relationships with the outside world, this identification forms the basis of all object-relationships. Future disturbances of these relationships frequently flow from a derangement in this identification, differing only in quality and degree. It is therefore concluded from these basic formations of Freud that a disturbance of the relationship to the outside world in deaf persons who develop psychosis may quite possibly be based upon such a disturbance of identification with the object.

Psychoanalytical research with regard to the manner in which different objects and events of the outside world are experienced and thus identified by the individual have shown that the element of movement plays a role of great importance, a point made by Freud in his paper, "Wit and Its Relation to the Unconscious." He proves here that we continuously identify ourselves unconsciously below the threshold of perception with the movement of objects which we notice in the outside world. Perception of object-movement is, therefore, an important factor for our relationship with the outside world.

According to Wallenberg in his stimulating paper, "On the Relation of Hearing to Space and Motion,"[9] this perception of object-movement is brought about partially by the visual sense, and our reaction to it may be ambivalent. Another important factor for the perception of movement seems to be the auditory sense independent of the vestibular apparatus. Hearing, in this sense, mediates spatial impressions as well as movement through consciously and unconsciously perceived sounds.

It can be asserted therefore by summarizing the studies of Wallenberg, that lack of hearing will lead to diminished perception of motion of the object-world, thus disturbing the possibility of identification. The concept of a "silent and motionless world" in this sense becomes identical with that of a "dead world." This concept when severely distorted can lead to psychosis or depression unless substitution through other senses takes place.

The numerous acoustic sensations from the outside world which we experience consciously and unconsciously help to give us the conception of movement in three-dimensional space by reason both of their spatial character and their slowness of transportation. In music, for instance, both space and motion are for the most part harmoniously perceived, and thus the identification with this "movement in unlimited space" may be complete and without ambivalence. On the other hand, a sudden complete silence creates in many persons a fear and a feeling of uncertainty, since an important medium of relationship with space and objects is abruptly withdrawn.

From the above assumptions, it can be stated that for the deaf the recognition of space and motion is disturbed in the sense that the connection between objects and the individual has been disturbed, while the individual's ability to identify himself with them has been lost or at least has been rendered difficult. This being so, the world of the deaf easily becomes motionless or "static."

Freud has stated that psychotic manifestations represent the attempt to restore order within the person and to reestablish relations with the outside world. To this end, auditory hallucinations become one of the many chaotic efforts used to regain connection with reality and so introduce movement to the static environment through hearing. The more fortunate of those afflicted with impaired hearing usually find a means of connection with the outside world through other senses. But for those suffering from serious hearing defects or total deafness, this distorted identification with the dead world often leads to deep depression, even to suicide.

In summary then, the ear, apart from its anatomical relationship to the body, serves a definite purpose in psychic life. Symbolically it plays a double role as a *receiver* of sound and as a *perceiver* of words and situations. It serves passively as the receptor of stimuli over auditory pathways; actively in the process of listening.

References

1. Joost A. M. Meerloo: *Conversation and Communication.* New York, International Universities Press, Inc., 1952, p. 18.
2. *Ibid.,* p. 123.
3. H. G. Wells, J. S. Huxley, and G. P. Wells: *The Science of Life.* New York, The Literary Guild, 1934, pp. 121-122.
4. S. R. Silverman: "Hard of Hearing Children." In H. Davis: *Hearing and Deafness.* New York, Rinehart, 1947, pp. 352-366.
5. Leo Kanner: *Child Psychiatry.* Springfield, Illinois, Charles C Thomas, Publisher, 1942, p. 32.
6. D. A. Ramsdell: "The Psychology of the Hard of Hearing and Deafened Adult." In H. Davis: *Hearing and Deafness.* New York, Rinehart, 1947, pp. 392-418.
7. Peter Hobart Knapp: "The Ear, Listening and Hearing." *Journal of the American Psychoanalytic Association,* Vol. I, No. 4, Oct. 1953, pp. 672-689.
8. Otto Isakower: "On the Exceptional Position of the Auditory Sphere." *International Journal of Psychoanalysis,* XX, pp. 3-4.

9. M. Wallenberg: "On the Relation of Hearing to Space and Motion." *The Psychiatric Quarterly*, Vol. 17, No. 4, p. 663.

10. A. Gesell and F. Ilg: *The Child from Five to Ten.* New York, Harper & Bros., 1946.

Listening with the Inner Ear

(*Listening to Ourselves*)

Talk to a man about himself and he will listen for hours.
—Disraeli

Most of us like to hear ourselves talk. Perhaps this is true because no matter what else we think, we are actually talking about ourselves. Yet this urge to talk leads to so much emptiness and meaningless chatter that it would be most illuminating were it possible to stand on the sidelines and listen to ourselves.

Nevertheless there are periods in our lives when we are overwhelmed by an awareness of inner conflict, loneliness, a sense of isolation; when the feelings we are experiencing cannot be expressed in ordinary conversation. At such times the need for privacy and the dread of exposing our innermost fears to others may compel us to withdraw from contact with others.

Silent contemplation over a prolonged period of time, however, makes for a lonely and unhealthy way of life. As humans we need to communicate with others so that we may reveal ourselves and identify with others. This urge to communicate, the awareness of being an entity, helps us to secure real contact with the world about us and find acceptance and understanding.

One of the dilemmas of modern man is to make himself both heard and understood. He has many ears and he speaks many languages. Yet there is always the barrier of words. We all want to communicate with each other, to develop common levels of agreement, but we need also to maintain our own individuality, to express our own personal feelings and opinions. We cannot attempt to understand or comprehend others until we learn to listen effectively to ourselves and so find the means of developing insight into life situations. A feeling *for* and *with* others cannot be experienced until we are able to put aside our selfish motives, prejudices and condemnations, and unless we try to understand each other through mutual identification. Only when this state of mutual relationship is reached can the individual integrate himself into other social formations.

In order to communicate with ourselves we need not necessarily remain alone. A good listener will serve as a mirror on which to cast the image of our real selves. This is what takes place in the therapeutic relationship with a psychiatrist. He listens not only to our words but to the hidden meanings behind our language. He becomes a sympathetic and understanding ear into which we pour our difficulties. He gives us an opportunity to *hear* ourselves talk. In this transmission he offers us the chance to talk freely, to listen to our deepest thoughts and hidden impulses and so to achieve a productive form of self-communication.

You can only communicate to yourself and to others what you feel and believe and accept in yourself. Those who feel they *should* communicate in pure form rather than in terms of what they actually are, can easily give false impressions which will transmit erroneous and distorted messages. Every speaker inevitably talks from within himself and, unavoidably, about himself and his innermost feelings.

Speech is a stimulis to both the listener and the speaker. In the listener, words may arouse feelings, emotions, ideas, action. Thus the listener too becomes excited, lonely, sad, happy, glad, fearful or depressed to the same degree that what we say and the way we express it frightens, saddens or excites us. The content and manner of our

33

utterances, the quality of our voice, emphasis, intensity and pitch of our speech, can all arouse feelings of varying intensity. Speech can incite feelings of love or anger, place us on the defensive, make us fearful to the point of withdrawal, or impel us to attack with anger or to embrace with love. Thus the *way* we talk and listen has a powerful influence not only on ourselves but on others.

In a strict sense whenever a person speaks, he does so to himself. Others may listen to his words and constitute themselves an audience. They may want to believe that the speaker is talking specifically to them. The speaker may also give this illusory impression, but essentially in what he says and to whom, he is actually communicating only with himself.

Of the speaker-listener relationship, L. E. Travis writes: "The speaker-listener interaction is the matrix of society. Speech is the leading character in the drama of interpersonal relationships. The speaker is an actor and the listener is an audience. Regardless of the part the speaker may think he is playing, in a way and to a degree he is always playing himself. And to the act the listener always responds. Sometimes more, sometimes less, sometimes painfully, sometimes joyfully, sometimes feelingly, sometimes intellectually, one's listening and viewing audience invariably responds. And in that response the speaker sees his own reflection. What he sees may not be true of him. It may be distorted by the form and quality of the listener's reflecting surfaces. Unintentionally, the speaker may arouse hate or fear or love in another. To his surprise, the speaker may see himself reflected as a hateful creature, or a fearful monster, or a lovable character."[1]

Man as a Symbolizing Animal

We as humans can only speak or listen in terms of our own self-created images and with whatever symbols we develop within ourselves. We learn to speak and listen without conscious effort and, as we relate interdynamically with the world about us, our speech assumes a special character and identity of its own. Depending on our own individual life experiences, needs, education, beliefs and attitudes, our modes of communication assume their own form, shape and purpose.

Man alone has the gift of a speaking language. As he emerged from the solitude of the prehistoric void into the complexity of modern society, he had more and more need to resort to symbols and in order to communicate and relate with the world about him, he found it necessary to seek for more workable tools. Most important of these was the creation of words and general concepts which we today call abstractions. With these man discovered that he could take the memory of past experiences, relate them to the experiences of the present and attempt to prognosticate what would happen in the future. But in order to make this a more effective process, he found that he must also learn how to listen and how to reflect.

Man's abstract attitude gives him the added capacity for making mental blueprints of intended actions, thus enabling him to plan ahead. With such an ability he can adopt certain patterns for the execution of future moves. His ears will be selective, discriminative, able to shift the patterns when necessary, and so to make a choice. Ultimately, the more astute this abstract attitude of his becomes and the more man's listening apparatus becomes specialized, the more will he be able to distinguish between essential and nonessential aspects of a given situation, between figure and background, and between similarity and identity.

One of the most valuable mental tools created by man is the symbol. Without it he might not have been able to communicate efficiently with his fellow man. As natural outgrowth of his need to communicate his individual opinions and feelings, he developed speech as a means of establishing social contact. It is true that animals do vocalize and communicate through sound and bodily movement, but only the human animal has the ability to speak, to be selective and be understood as to thought and meaning. As an individual, he may choose to speak, to be silent, or to listen.

Had we not created symbols, we should have had to deal directly with *things* instead of being able to express our ideas and feelings through *words*. But through the spoken and written word, man's traditions have been preserved and passed along from generation to generation. Without speech or the capacity to hear, we should perforce have reverted to the level of the beasts, and the whole structure of society and civilization would have crumbled and disintegrated.

Speech as a form of symbolic transformation gives meaning to life's experiences. With speech we streamline our communications, understand each other more clearly and make social interaction possible. In listening to each other, we interpret and re-interpret experience. Language is projective. We use symbols to describe events, to make statements about ourselves, and to give meaning and continuity to experience. Thus man draws from the *past*, interrelates with—and in—the *present*, and makes ready for the *future*.

Symbolizing is a basic bodily process in the human being. Susanne Langer in *Philosophy in a New Key* says, in effect, that it is of the nature of man that he must transform all his experiences into words, or colored patches, melodies, bronze statues or other patterns of symbols. He does this as naturally as he eats, drinks or makes love. Man, continues Dr. Langer, has a basic need for using, manipulating, arranging, recalling, inventing, changing, expressing and responding generally to and with symbols of various kinds. The symbolizing process thus becomes a natural outgrowth of man's development and living.

Symbols in general also unify the varied experiences of the individual members of a social group through the associations they are capable of evoking. Religious symbolism, for example, is tremendously meaningful to many people in different ways.

The process of symbolization helps us to face and to listen to irrational and frightening natural phenomena close to our everyday living by using symbols which make them appear more concrete and realistic, hence less threatening. In this sense, the symbolizing process aids us in temporarily "shutting off our ears" to unbearable conflicting situations, and thus protects us from anxiety.

It is my contention, stated in my book *Your Speech Reveals Your Personality*, that the symbolizing process is a fundamental aspect of the whole personality. Man creates symbols not only to communicate verbally with others and thus establish interpersonal relationships, but also to serve as an integrating process within himself. In his attempts to find himself in his search for inner truth and psychic unity, he of necessity creates a personal language of his own, with verbal and non-verbal symbols peculiar and specific to his own way of life. His greatest difficulty will arise, of course, in his need to find word-symbols he can understand, utilize and experience which at the same time will enable him to communicate outwardly with others on mutual levels of comprehension and agreement.

The concept or image a person has of himself is dependent: a) on the factors belonging to his structural being, and b) on his state of psychic health. This last factor is highly proportionate to one's inner sense of comprehension and perception, and here listening plays a most important role.

When perceiving, we have a degree of inner choice or selectivity. From birth man by means of his "inner ear" adapts himself to the best of his ability to the world around him. He attempts to create and choose those symbols with which he can efficiently relate to himself and to others. Accordingly he must learn a system of symbolization and language if he wishes to participate within a given group. He must also learn, through the impact of mass communication, how to interpret and use messages so that they can be accepted by and shared with others.

Situations have different meanings for different people and vary from time to time. For instance, we begin with a happening—something is going on. We observe it. In reality no two people can perceive the same thing in exactly the same way because: (1) our sense organs function somewhat differently no matter how similar their basic functions may be; (2) our previous life experiences are somewhat different no matter how similar they might appear to be and previous experiences influence and make a significant difference in what and how we perceive; and (3) our points of observation cannot be the same because no two observers or listeners can occupy the same place at the same time. Therefore, of all the various aspects of the happening which we may consciously notice or hear, we will select different aspects and with different feelings.

An individual can only perceive and listen in proportion to his relative state of psychic health. The closer a person is to himself and the more energies he tends to direct toward health and away from neurosis, the more realistic will be his picture of himself and his environment. The concept of one's self is never simon pure but will always contain rational and irrational aspects. Also, in the process of living or integrating the individual is always symbolizing and abstracting. The more irrational a person's concept is of himself, the less he will be able to perceive healthily and the more he will tend to equate words with things, to select indiscriminately, and to project his own confused feelings and emotions in his communications.

When our symbolizing mechanism becomes faulty, we function ineffectively and as a result we listen with "confused and disturbed ears." The *verbal world* which comes to us mainly through words as opposed to the world we know through our own experience makes for a habitual confusion of symbols. We no longer depend upon our own resources or abilities to perceive correctly. Instead we resort to the outside and to others to give personal meaning to our lives. We lose our inner discriminating capacity, we fear to make choices we like, and we tend to live through other people's thoughts, feelings and beliefs. We listen thus not through our own selves but through other people's ears.

The Feedback Mechanism

We usually talk about the speaker and listener as though they were two different persons. In a dynamic sense, it would be much more effective to evaluate them as part of a single communicative process, as though they were one and the same.

Norbert Wiener, who has attracted widespread interest in the science of the transfer of information which he calls *cybernetics*, made the following penetrating observation in his book *The Human Use of Human Beings:* "Speech is a joint game between the talker and the listener against the forces of confusion." Wiener, a mathematician, systematized the theory of communicative engineering. His formulations of the notion of feedback and their application to social behavior gave us the theoretical foundations for the understanding of corrective communication.

The foremost criterion of successful communication is the presence of these circuits which provide a means for relaying back to the original sender the effects that an utterance has had upon others. Effective communications occurs when two or more participants reach mutual levels of agreement and when they are ready and curious enough to work incessantly toward further improvement of the facilities for feedback.

Listening plays a most important role in the correction of information and the stabilizing of these circuits. For example, a listener's response to a speaker's statement—its clarity, distinctness, relevance and timing—will often be more important than the actual subject matter and its formulations. For healthy relationships to take place between people, we must learn to approach one another with tact, tolerance and consideration. If, however, we cease to listen to ourselves or to others and block attempts to learn and bring information up to date, communication between individuals will eventually break down. Successful communication depends primarily upon both the ability of a speaker to transmit messages in such a way that his statements can be correctly interpreted and on the listener's proficiency in understanding these same statements. This will depend largely upon the feedback circuits and the manner in which they are used.

There are two general kinds of feedback: the internal feedback, which comes from sources within the speaker himself; and the external feedback which comes from sources outside the speaker. The internal feedback is at work when the speaker is being reflective about something he has just said, while the external feedback operates when the speaker becomes alert and sensitive to the reactions of his listeners to what he has said. These two circuits necessarily affect each other at the same or different intervals to that which is going on. They are closely interrelated and depend strongly upon each other. Even if no other persons are present, the speakers' reflections on what he has just said or thought is influenced to some degree by his past experiences and by his consideration of possible future experiences. So when we say that there are two kinds of feedback, we do so, according to Wendell Johnson, "with the realization, of course, that while they might be distinguished, one from the other, they cannot possibly be disentangled. As his own listener, every speaker attends as best he can as though with the ears of a multitude."[2]

If we are properly attuned in our listening, we can formulate and reply selectively and positively to one or more aspects of a message. For instance, in the crucial formative years of a child's development, a parent, either by selectively responding to the statements of the child or by exposing the child to statements of his own, imperceptibly directs and influences the communication system of the child. Selective feedback is therefore of utmost importance in parent-child communication and parents who are not good listeners frequently produce disturbed feedback patterns in their children. In the adult, in contrast to the child, disturbances in feedback patterns are different not so much in content as in quality, degree and complexity of replies.

Listening with Static

In addition to disturbances in the feedback mechanism, we also listen poorly or with "static" when we are not properly attuned to ourselves. Because of difficulties which we have created within ourselves, we put artificial barriers before our capacity to perceive healthily and thus block any real form of communication. At these times, our listening posts become further apart and messages from the outside and from our inner voices become inaudible and confused. The more hazy and vague our listening becomes, the finer and more calibrated a tuning mechanism is necessary. We need greater energies to concentrate and pay attention to what is being communicated to us. To comprehend better during these static periods, it is essential that we adjust our hearing to higher wave length frequencies, and to concentrate the harder so that we may remain an active part of the listening exchange.

When our listening is interfered with, it also becomes more difficult to search within ourselves for the real truths.

Most listening is subjective. Psychological evidence demonstrates that too often we hear and experience only that which interests us and stimulates our inner feelings. We listen mainly in terms of our primary needs, translating into our own language and words that which we perceive and conceptualize. A well trained stenographer, for instance, absorbs out of the many words pictures she receives only for those she understands, whereas those she does not comprehend inhibit her work.

We are all familiar, for instance, with the everyday expressions: a child, told to "listen to his elders," is expected to heed and obey; a "hearing" is a review by a tribunal; to "turn a deaf ear" is to ignore an ethical claim or threat; an adolescent child who feels coerced and pressured by his parents may say that he was going to pull off his ears—"so I won't have to hear the grownups and do what they say."

Many of us, when conflicted, impose upon ourselves inner dictates concerning what we feel we should be able to do, to be, to know, and various taboos on how and what we should not be. These dictates usually become compulsive, indiscriminate and inexorably felt, what Karen Horney calls "the tyranny of the should."

When tense or anxious, many listeners place demands upon themselves which, though understandable, are altogether too difficult and too rigid. Illusions and self-idealizations drive them relentlessly toward perfection in all areas, including listening. Characteristically, these demands are destructive and unfeasible and show a complete *disregard for the conditions* under which they could be fulfilled. The "tyranny of the should" operates with a supreme *disregard for the person's own psychic condition*, for what he can feel or do as he is at present.

The disturbed listener thus puts distractions in the path of his listening by making impossible demands on his delicate hearing apparatus. He tends to rely on his intellect for most of his life resources and so listens chiefly with his brain. It is essential to him that his hearing mechanism must *never fail him*. He demands of himself push-button action for listening to and remembering all facts, knowledge, wording, vocabulary and detailed data. If he should fail and listen incorrectly or should not approximate these heights of intellectual know-it-all, he will feel—irrationally—that he will be judged inadequate, ignorant and stupid.

Still further, the ineffectual listener is constantly on the defensive against being caught in error, and if he is criticized, disagreed with, or if any of his shortcomings are exposed by others, he is either roused to anger, defiance, abused feelings, or he is reduced to a silent sulkiness. He must never be judged wrong, for in his sense of the word, this implies weakness and he then experiences what he dreads most—the feeling of being stupid. This worship of intellect and the over-emphasis on being always the alert, keen and intelligent listener becomes so intensified at times that it predominates and excludes many other attitudes and vital areas in life.

The poor listener places an overemphasis on the spoken word with all of its intellectual colorings and too little emphasis on nonverbal content. He listens to words as though they were realities or facts in themselves. For the insecure listener, the spoken word carries an effect of tremendous impact. Believing that words assure him mastery and control in most situations, such a person finds it imperative to measure his words and to use them with utter care and caution lest a careless word bring about a disturbance or calamity. For him there is little recognition of his "belonging" to his words or of inner choice, freedom or discrimination in the communication situation. Listening therefore becomes a "should" and is filled with connotations of perfection, mastery and intellectual brilliancy.

1. THE INTELLECTUAL OR LOGICAL TYPE OF LISTENER

Of those who may be considered poor listeners, the *"logical"* or *intellectual* type listens mostly with his head and denies his real feelings in a situation. He listens only to what he wants to hear, blotting out larger areas of reality. His vanity and egocentricity compel him to think solely of himself. He does not acknowledge the intent of the other person, nor does he care whether that person has received his message in the way it was intended. Being interested mainly in rational appraisal, he tends to neglect emotional and nonverbal aspects of living. He is inclined, according to Ruesch, "to operate at the intrapersonal level, regardless of the situation. His evaluation is selectively geared to the interpretation of verbal statements of others. He prefers to deal with syntactic and semantic rather than with pragmatic aspects."[3] He is not interested in what impact his statements may produce upon others, nor is he capable of viewing the effect that the statement of another person may have upon him. He listens in terms of categories, making certain that what he listens to does not disturb his inner peace or systematic order. In any communicative exchange he rarely interferes with his speaker, listening as he speaks, waiting always for the moment when he himself can talk and the other listen.

This listener's fear of close relations with others also compels him consciously to choose and establish contact with those suitable and receptive to his own needs. He listens with little concern for the speaker and blots out many of his real feelings by creating a distance between himself and others. This he attempts to accomplish by seeking refuge in the stratospheric levels of his imagination where he can protect himself from listening to anything that can be a possible threat to his omnipotence.

44

2. THE EMOTIONAL OR OVER-ANXIOUS LISTENER

The *emotional* listener is one who, as opposed to the logical listener, listens almost entirely with his feelings and too little with his head. His over-anxious make-up accelerates his level of tension and excitation to the point which exceeds the capacity for reception, evaluation, or transmission of that particular person. The resultant effect is a jamming and disorganization of the communication network.

A listener of this type because of his fear of feeling anxiety or being involved in conflict attempts to accelerate or slow down his hearing mechanism to suit his own neurotic attitudes. What ensues, however, is that in his chaotic and compulsive actions, he becomes more defenseless against the bombardment of those stimuli which disturb his communication network and a vicious circle is formed. His fear of listening to disturbing or alarming messages disorganizes his listening capacity to the extent of jamming up the entire communication network. He cannot listen effectively, his relations with others become disturbed, and in his further struggle to remedy the situation, he becomes the more anxious and chaotic.

In his attempts to restore psychic unity, the over-anxious listener may resort to interpersonal relations to alleviate his fear and anxiety. However, since a person of this sort places his main emphasis on reducing the number or the intensity of the stimuli, he will often reduce the number of incoming messages by curtailing social contact with others. In so doing he abandons the only anxiety-reducing mechanism at his disposal. What he does not perceive is that this flood of disturbing stimuli which he fears originates mainly from *within* himself rather than from the outside.

This type listener uses so much of his energies avoiding conflict-provoking situations that he has little energy left for constructive use. In his multiple, self-created, compulsive attempts to escape from pain and frustration, he tends also to disregard the gratification of more vital needs, which will lead to an impoverishment of experience and a denial of pleasure. His listening becomes fixed at a primitive level as words are equated with things, having for the most part interpretations and meanings of danger and anxiety. Communication with others deteriorates and messages are frequently misinterpreted because his attention is focused on the presence or absence of alarm rather than on the total context and the full meaning of the statement.

Listening with Attuned Ears

When we listen with attuned ears, we concentrate on keeping our listening paths open and readied for signals which originate both from within ourselves and from others. To do so effectively, it is essential that we sharpen both our "inner and outer ears" in an effort to remove those distractions and disturbances which ordinarily interfere with harmonious listening.

Many of us in listening distort the true meanings of things because we fear intimacy with others and make evaluations on surface externals and prejudices. We make snap judgments based on looks, on clothes and on other physical exterior details instead of on more meaningful values.

Few people *really* listen to each other, primarily because they are self-centered or are intensely diverted by what they *see*. They are so accustomed to learning about others through their eyes that they do not listen on more intimate levels. To listen with purpose, it is essential that we not arrive at impulsive conclusions or deductions through words or externals. Instead we should learn to view the world about us less through our eyes and more through our feelings and our inherent capacity to listen. In so doing, we shall understand more of the implied meanings behind words, names, labels. Then, as we relate more intimately with the world we live in, its complexities will grow less mysterious and confused and we shall be able to communicate more effectively with truthful meaning and a sense of responsibility, mutual rapport and understanding.

Robert Barnett, present president of the American Foundation for the Blind, in a recent interview with Mike Wallace gave a most vivid explanation of why he thought most people are afraid of the blind: "Actually the almost stark intimacy required by the blind—the direct, intense listening to each other—is what frightens people who can see . . . They are obliged to come out from behind facades. They can't hide behind their masks . . . their false smiles . . . their hair-dos . . . their Brooks Brothers suits. They know, unconsciously, that the blind man will penetrate all these camouflages and get directly to *them*. This, I think, is what underlies the fear."

Many people do not wish to understand others or to be understood. They are satisfied too quickly with the periphery and externals of things, fearing any kind of deep personal involvement. They like talking and listening only if the conversation does not go too deep. They are less interested in personal satisfaction and only want answers to their questions. They insist on such rigid two-valued dichotomies as right-or-wrong, black-or-white, all-or-none. They listen to others, absorbing noises and sounds with too little concern for effect, content or truth. They nod and shake their heads compulsively, wanting to give the impression of being intelligent, but denying their real problems. They hide behind the facade of having fully comprehended, yet they leave the situation empty-handed. They have achieved little insight, real understanding or self-growth. It is this kind of empty communication that leads to a scarcity of real human contact in the world. Too many of us behave like automatons, relating mechanically to each other. We are deaf and mute when somebody else tries to speak. We listen with "tin ears."

In listening effectively, we must attune ourselves to our own as well as to other people's wave lengths. The truth cannot be achieved by stopping our ears against the sounds of our own inner voices. Real inner peace is not achieved by blocking out the awareness of conflict, pain, struggle or disquietude. All are essential and realistic parts of living. We must instead open our ears and permit ourselves to become involved with the world about us as *it actually is*, not as we feel *it should be*. We must realize that our true reflections as human beings come into light only insofar as we have the courage to face ourselves. This necessitates not only talking freely to ourselves but *wholly* listening to others. We shall then lean less toward accepting answers as finalities and will progress more toward a realistic finding of the truth.

References

1. Lee Edward Travis (Editor): *Handbook of Speech Pathology.* New York, Appleton-Century-Crofts, Inc., 1957, p. 967.
2. Wendell Johnson: *Your Most Enchanted Listener.* New York, Harper & Brothers, 1957, p. 174.
3. Jurgen Ruesch: *Disturbed Communication.* New York, Norton & Co., 1957, p. 127.

Listening with a Receptive Ear

(Listening to Others)

Speak, in order that I may see you—
—Socrates

Each word expressed by the speaker has its own individual meaning, but it also has a private picture which only the listener receives. As a rule we see or hear only what we *believe* we are perceiving at the moment. We create our own visual and auditory images to suit our individual needs and existing motivations, and frequently what we envision is not what is seen by others nor is it the actual object of our seeing. As Wendell Johnson puts it, "we see what isn't there at all: the believing that is seeing."[1]

The spoken word is a powerful and hypnotic motivator. A speaker with a fiery delivery and an ability to persuade masses easily suggests, excites, exhilarates and even incites intense feelings in those who listen to him. So it is that a powerful speaker like Evangelist Billy Graham is able to persuade thousands of those who flock to hear him crusade to change their way of life.

When listening, we rarely question or stop to assess the truth of what we hear. We are too prone to open our ears to mass suggestion and too willing to mold ourselves in the group image. We allow ourselves to be excited, sad, joyous or angry as we react to what the speaker wants us to feel. We listen and react primarily by habit and suggestion. We become compulsive listeners.

49

As habitual listeners we automatically follow the statements and facts of others without bothering to use our own evaluative faculties. In certain emotionally colored situations we become easily swayed by words alone and allow ourselves to be influenced by the speaker's voice, its hypnotic and trance-like quality, the intonations and the rhythm of the sounds he utters. At such times we are unable to evaluate meaningfully but communicate in relation to the degree to which we are impressed and affected. Communicative situations of this sort bear the quality of hypnotic seances in which words act as vehicles for transferring emotion and feeling. Their specific meaning is secondary.

The power of sound has always been greater than the power of sense. Not the right argument but the right sound and word have influence. Most of us prefer to be impressed and affected rather than convinced by logic.

Who of us, for example, does not remember that night of terror and folly, October 30, 1938, when Orson Welles over the radio persuaded several million Americans that their country was being invaded by flame-spitting Martians who looked like snakes and stood as tall as bears? At 8 P.M. on that particular evening, about six million people across the United States heard the following announcement on their radios: "The Columbia Broadcasting System and its affiliated stations present Orson Welles and the Mercury Theatre of the Air in *The War of the Worlds*, by H. G. Wells."

This announcement was followed by a weather report and dance music. Suddenly the dance music was interrupted by a "flash" news story: "A series of gas explosions has just been noted on the planet Mars," said the announcement. The broadcast went on to report that a meteor had landed near Princeton, New Jersey, killing fifteen hundred persons. A few minutes later, however, came a further report: it was no meteor but a metal cylinder out of which poured Martian creatures armed for a death ray attack upon the earth.

Halfway through the hour long program, two announcements were made which clearly indicated that what people were hearing was only a fiction story. The same announcement was made at the program's conclusion. And at least 60 per cent of all the radio stations carrying the program interrupted the play to make the same statement. Yet about a million people did not hear these announcements. Only the single word "invasion" caught their ears and they were gripped with fear and panic.

There were those, wrote Harriet Van Horne years later in reviewing a television drama based on the event, ". . . the simple ones *who believeth every word*, who loaded their rifles, packed some provender, bundled their sleepy tots into the family jalopy and fled to the hills."[2] In this Studio One "re-enactment of the now famous episode," we saw how blind, unreasoning fear overtook a baby-sitter, a poker game, a trio of toughs in a bar, and a timid old man in a furnished room, and even a listener present in the radio studio reacted to the report of the snake-like men emerging from the space cylinder. The entire program was a most graphic example of how easily words, sounds and drama can inflame thousands. It also dramatically illustrated how poorly millions of Americans *listen*.

Listening to Persuasive Speech

The art of persuasion is another powerful weapon for influencing and motivating the average listener. Among the oldest of the arts, it is one which we unconsciously attempt to cultivate within ourselves. To that end we begin to expose our children at an early age to dubious concepts of the world we live in and to all sorts of influences through the powerful media of television, radio, the comics and the movies. From the moment he begins to listen and read, the child is confronted by such periodicals as Mad Magazine and the comics. Throughout his later development, he is taught to believe that words carry a tremendous impact. We learn that words are capable of assuring us mastery and control in most life situations. We discover too that through misevaluated interpretations, man has given magical properties to words which in actuality do not exist. Our language has thus become a personal interpretation of our inner feelings instead of a true representation of the objective realities.

In our present culture we have grown increasingly persuasion-minded. Our tendency is to seek means for arriving at compromise and for interrelating with each other by persuasion rather than by force. Thomas Mann once wrote that "speech is civilization," another way of saying that words used for purposes of discussion and persuasion are the most civilized tools with which to settle differences and attempt to live realistically with each other.

In a broad sense, persuasion is any form of discourse that influences thought, feelings or conduct. "It is surely true," says Oliver in his excellent book, *The Psychology of Persuasive Speech*, "that no speech that truly informs listeners can avoid influencing their judgment and hence their future behavior."[3] In persuasive discourse, the speaker makes a calculated effort to change the personality orientation of his listeners by continually vibrating their eardrums. His ultimate purpose is to render his audience different—in belief, in attitude, in feeling, in conduct—as a direct result of his words. In achieving this end, his most useful weapon is his belief that most people are credulous by way of the ear.

Too many of us are too quick to accept as fact the utterances of politicians, lobbyists, college professors, radio and television commentators and super-salesmen. We often lack the ability to be selective, discriminating or critical of the spoken word. We fall prey to the cunning

52

way in which a persuasive speaker seduces us with his words and so directs our entire attention to his oratory, thereby persuading us, as we listen, to accept his views as though they were gospel.

Wendell Johnson, in discussing the seriousness of this problem, goes even further: "As speakers, men have become schooled in the arts of persuasion; and without the counter-art of listening a man can be persuaded— even by his words—to eat foods that ruin the liver, to abstain from killing flies, to vote away his right to vote, and to murder his fellows in the name of righteousness. The art of listening holds for us the desperate hope of withstanding the spreading ravages of commercial, nationalistic and ideological persuasion."[4]

Another important role of persuasive speaking is to sway the listener's emotions. Aristotle once said that "persuasion may come through the hearers, when the speech stirs their emotions . . ." Three hundred years later, Cicero wrote that "all the emotions of the mind which nature has given to man must be intimately known; for all the force and art of speaking must be employed in allaying or exciting the feelings of those who listen." The opinions of these ancient rhetoricians are still well supported today.

There is no doubt that in most situations emotions, in one way or another, play an important part. Whenever something is experienced as close or important to us, we become emotionally involved. Should we respond to something only with our heads and deny our feelings, we would be reduced to the level of automatons. In general a speaker attempts to impress his audience through his personal appearance, behavior, manner, voice, diction and the general impact of his personality. All these factors are involved in the presentation and delivery of the speech.

Persuasion also, to a considerable degree, depends upon personality. Authority or leadership in any given situation gives an individual a marked advantage in the persuasive process. The very fact that, culture-wise, so many of us are accustomed to accepting blindly the words of the so-called "authorities" and rarely question their validity helps such speakers in persuading their listeners. The persuasive speaker can spellbind his audiences and hold them in the hollow of his hand. Pigors says in *Leadership or Domination*, "Followers respect their leader's superiority in certain traits, aspirations and judgments, because they recognize their traits as their own,"[3] and so makes the point that the persuasive strength of the speaker comes mainly from the nature of his audience. In this way both speaker and listener relate to and motivate each other inter-dynamically.

The persuasive speaker uses a variety of techniques to get people to listen to and accept his own self-imposed views. He seeks to so influence listeners that they will give up their own self-evaluative and critical faculties, thus becoming the parrot-like and helpless victims of his charming words. In so doing, he is acting in the belief that if people can be made to think quickly, compulsively and to "jump to conclusions," they will accept most anything as the truth.

One specific area where techniques in the art of persuasion are well planned and masterfully used to provoke a sympathetic ear is in the use of propaganda. Aldous Huxley once said that it is the function of propaganda to enable people to do in cold blood things that they could otherwise do only in the heat of passion. The propagandist is less concerned with direct emotions than he is with persuading his audience that what he says contains more than the truths of man-made conventions. His emphasis is mainly in the direction of persuading his listeners that the propaganda message is an objective statement rather than a metacommunicative message. The ideas or facts of propaganda, be that in the form of a film, play or magazine article, are accentuated as "typical" and—in a sense—objective truth.

Hitler's pronouncements were a graphic illustration of the old saying, that if a lie is big enough and is told often enough, many people will believe it. Much of the propaganda emanating from communistic dictatorships is obviously based upon this same premise, the primary aim being to initiate desired action patterns in listeners and to block off and eliminate others which might interfere with the desired aim of the propaganda.

In a totalitarian setting, the word acts as the most powerful tool. Vocabulary becomes a dictated set of words used not in the service of communication and conversation but rather in the service of party propaganda. To again quote Meerloo: "In the same way as verbosity is used by the individual to suffocate the free mind of the listener, verbocracy is used to suffocate the free minds of its followers. The empty word, as well as every human expression and communication, is under the control of a magic center. A calculated strategy of semantic confusion is used to blackmail man's intellectual laziness."[5]

In listening to propaganda, we are being conditioned to absorb beliefs others wish us to hear and accept half-truths or distorted facts colored so as to appear as familiar and normal, and our ears hear only those messages which the speaker wants us to with little or no dependence upon our own critical abilities. And since we are not impelled to question or understand what is being set forth, we either *do not hear* or *we believe we have heard something quite different from what was actually said.*

Messages for the most part find their meaning and significance in the responses made to them by listeners. In *Mein Kampf* Hitler explained why he chose to use spoken rather than written propaganda for the purpose of addressing the Nazi mass meetings:

55

An orator receives continuous guidance from his audience, enabling him to correct his lecture, since he can measure all the time on the countenances of his hearers the extent to which they are successful in following his arguments intelligently and whether his words are producing the effect he desires, whereas the writer has no acquaintance with his readers. Hence he is unable to prepare his sentences with a view to addressing a definite crowd of people, sitting in front of his eyes, but he is obliged to argue in general terms.

Supposing that an orator observes that his hearers do not understand him, he will make his explanation so elementary and clear that every single one must take it in; if he feels that they are incapable of following him, he will build up his ideas carefully and slowly until the weakest member has caught up, again, once he senses that they seem not to be convinced that he is correct in his arguments, he will repeat them over and over again with fresh illustrations and himself state their unspoken objections; he will continue thus until the last group of the opposition show him by their behavior and play of expression that they have capitulated to his demonstration of the case.[6]

The Need to be Heard

Just as urgently as we desire to be persuaded and influenced by others, we also have a strange need to be heard. Shakespeare said this poetically in his

"All the world's a stage,
And all the men and women merely players."

Everyone in one way or another wants to be heard. There are those talkers who, in their urgency to be listened to at any cost, become perpetual bores. A bore has been defined as someone who talks when you want him to listen. In Senator (Texas) Lyndon Johnson's office is a sign which says pointedly: *You Ain't Learning Nothin' When You're Talkin'*. In other words, it would be well—

in this area—if we concentrated on what we intended to say and were also alert and attentive in listening to others.

In our listening, it isn't the words themselves that lead to possible misunderstanding but rather our preconceived notion and attitude toward the speaker and his words and the communicative situation. For speech to be effective there must be mutual areas of agreement and compromise between the speaker and the listener. Growth in the communicative act can only occur when both participants feel satisfaction and pleasure and so reach productive levels of understanding and acknowledgment.

When listening effectively, we tend to relate to the speaker as a whole rather than to his words or sounds. In every listening we strive to be accepted, loved, and to recognize or find something of ourselves. Though we appear to be attentive and concentrating on the specific word, what we generally are affected by is the effect we have on each other at the specific time of communication. We seem to be more influenced by the intention *behind* the word than its actual contextural meaning. The fact that a handsome speaker with the most absurd and inconsequential communication will provoke a great feeling of enthusiasm and ecstasy in an infatuated young listener of the opposite sex shows that what is important and crucial here is the emotional impact at the time of listening.

In social conversation, the "togetherness" of our meeting and the *desire* to talk and be listened to become the primary factors; the subject matter is secondary. Much that happens in our day-to-day living is neither serious nor profound. Therefore it is not necessary that we always feel compelled to listen attentively or to think reflectively. So it is that coffee breaks, teas, club meetings, bull sessions, social dates of various kinds, offer a respite from pressures and tensions. It is this coming together through words— daily conversations, small talk, gossip and so on—and the meaning behind our listening that has given us an important medium of social contact with which to break through barriers of strangeness and create more intimate relationships among ourselves.

"All listening," says Meerloo, "is subjective, an inner translation into one's own language, and this function is accompanied by the interpretation of the spoken word."[6] The true meaning of a message is to be found not in the actual words themselves, but in the personal translations given to them by the speaker and the listener. And, in evaluating the entire process, it is essential to know that there is always a difference between the meaning of a message to be found in the speaker's words and the meaning of the same message to be discovered in the listener. This difference, which is usually so slight as not to be noticed, is often lost in the conversational exchange. However, if it does become obvious, it may create serious disturbances or even a breakdown in the communication process.

For effective communication between two people, there must be adequate feedback circuits and relays from listener to speaker. The speaker for his part must be properly receptive to this feedback and the listener effectively receptive to the speaker's subsequent revisings—if any. Both speaker and listener dynamically keep sending and receiving messages, decodifying as they go along, to a point where mutual understanding and acknowledgment are achieved.

At times, however, we listen to almost anything that supports our secret neurotic strivings. There are individuals who, in their urgency to appear "god-like" and omnipotent toward everyone, tend to direct all of their available energies toward absolute perfection when listening. They want at all costs to be impressively attentive and intelligent, to have a magnetic personality. As listeners, these people use their hearing ability not to listen effectively but rather to select out of context only such facts or situations as they can successfully exploit to impress, outsmart and outwit others. Like the compulsive speaker, they too must come up with the *right answers* at all times. In a sense, they listen primarily with their brains and rarely with their feelings. Their need to listen is foremost in the direction of intellectual know-it-all and brilliance. To give their speakers—or, more specifically, those whom they wish to impress—the feeling that they are constantly alert, enthusiastic and enlightened is a most important aspect of their listening.

When listening compulsively, we easily become tense and confused if we fear standing alone on our own self-evaluation and convictions, and instead choose to evaluate our worth and status through the opinions and assertions of others. If, in our inadequacy, we need to listen mainly through the ears of others in order to win them over to our side and gain their praise and recognition, then it follows that our listening will become disturbed. Only when we consider our own wishes or opinions, instead of compulsively needing to prove ourselves to others, will we learn to use our ears more spontaneously and effectively.

Non-Verbal Listening

What reaches us through words is only one side of the picture. There is also a "non-verbal" communication, expressed in the interplay of hidden gestures, feelings, bodily reactions, glances, etc., which is constantly going on in dynamic human beings. An awareness of both verbal and non-verbal facts is essential in order to arrive at a more complete understanding of human behavior.

Consider the silent and hidden interaction of feelings, thoughts and actions either of a conjectured or comprehensive nature which occurs between two or more persons in the subterranean communicative channels of language. Much of this is consciously heard. However it also comes to us through sight, touch and smell. Still other aspects are relayed to us by the process of intuition and through

59

unconsciously felt perceptions. We communicate every minute of the day with others and with the outside through "speaking gestures—i.e., peculiarities in gait and dress, a sense of touch in a handshake, mannerisms, glances or looks, skin condition and texture, color of eyes, lips, body build, and a multitude of similar characteristics.

The most minute movements—muscular twitchings in face or hands and movements of the ears or eyes—"speak" as clearly as words, and we constantly receive other neurodynamic stimuli which play a part in producing our impressions though we may not be conscious of noticing them. There are still other sounds or expressive movements that we understand without conscious perception really being at work in that understanding. Also there are certain vocal modulations—the particular pitch and timbre of a voice, a particular speech rhythm—which we may not consciously observe; and there are variations of tone, pauses and shifted accentuation so slight that they miss our ears and never reach the limits of conscious observation. Though we may not be wholly aware of these stimuli and characteristics, they nevertheless tell us a great deal about a person. Socrates once said: "Speak, in order that I may see you." Frequently a voice we hear, even when the speaker is not seen, may tell us more about him than if we were actually observing him. It is not the actual words spoken but what those words tell us about the speaker that is of ultimate importance.

Originally language was an instinctive utterance. Not until much later in time did it develop from an undifferentiated whole into a specific means of communication and the actual language of words take the place of gesture language. As the famous linguist, Sir Richard Paget, points out, the movements of the tongue originally imitated our various actions.

What goes on on the non-verbal, silent—or "unspeakable"—levels in relation to life facts can only be differentiated in terms of our individual reactions, orientations, needs and evaluations. The problem we have in not being able to demonstrate these non-verbal levels in direct and absolute representations is not necessarily one of inadequacy of words. We can always invent "adequate" words, but even the most ideal and structurally adequate language will not be the *things* or *feelings* themselves. Distortions in listening and speaking effectively occur usually because of our reluctance to accept *what is* and because of our inner anxieties, our tendency to create conflicts and apprehensions, idealizations and magical identities with words and symbols. In our further attempts to listen to and verbalize our feelings, actions, beliefs and emotions as we feel they *should be* rather than as they exist in *actual reality*, we necessarily are compelled to create and use a vocabulary of magic and imaginative identification which abounds in confused attitudes toward words and symbols.

One pitfall that is common when listening is the acceptance of most assumptions or inferences as truths. An inference may be defined as a statement of the unknown made on the basis of the known. We may *infer* a man's wealth or social position, for instance, from such cultural externals as the pretentiousness of his home, automobile, or clothes; we may *infer* from the noise of a human cry that a person is in some form of danger; we may *infer* from a man's bodily configuration the nature of his work; we may *infer* from a senator's vote on an economic bill his attitude toward small or large business. These inferences may be made on the basis of a wealth of previous experience with the subject matter or of no experience at all. For example, the inferences the trained psychiatrist makes about the prognosis of a person's state of mental health are much more accurate and truthful than any inferences made by the so-called "parlor analyst" who bases his facts on hearsay and irrational deductions. In short, inferences are generally statements about matters not directly known to the conscious mind, made on the basis of what has previously been observed, felt or experienced.

In relating to others in listening or talking, we are expressing our opinions, feelings, beliefs or awareness to the degree to which our thoughts or statements are projective representations of our own inner state of being at the particular time of expression. This process in itself is variable, flexible and dynamically changeable from person to person, object to object, and situation to situation. In both listening and in our verbal statements, we perceive facts mainly as they appear *to us* and in relation to our inner condition at the time. These perceptions are often expressed by such words as "it seems to me," "from my point of view," "as I see it, it appears thus and so," etc.

In disturbed listening, impressions between observers differ not so much in relation to the facts at hand, but in the use of different variable adjectives. For instance, the questions, was Jack Dempsey the greatest of champions or merely a good boxer in his prime and day?, which is the best form of relaxation—reading, golf, movies, tennis or radio?, or could Willy Mays outhit Ty Cobb in his prime?, usually result in aimless and fruitless debate. In such instances, verbal interchange between people leads to little productivity, since there can be no settlement of the question and they invariably result in emotional interplay which has very little connection with the issue at hand. If this insistence on "splitting hairs" persists, more and more superlative adjectives tend to be injected into the discussion and less and less agreement occurs and the situation will therefore end in confusion and discord. Were we to listen more without prejudice, criticism or condemnation and argue less without flaring emotions and fixed opinions of our own, we might then be able to communicate with each other with more meaningful purpose. An end result would be that we should leave the discussion better informed, more aware of things, and less one-sided and dogmatic than we were before the conversation began.

A second method by which we should be able to prevent conflicting issues in a discussion from becoming an argument is to move the talk from the level of judgment-making to more descriptive levels. In other words, instead of attempting to debate the issue of whether Ty Cobb or Willy Mays is the better hitter or fielder, it would be more constructive to discuss at length the individual qualities, attributed or accomplished actions of either or both the players involved.

By using objective facts as a basis for shared discussion, levels of agreement are more easily achieved, genuine understanding more easily reached, and the continuation of talk on healthier planes of evaluation is more readily accessible.

Listening with Humility

Charles P. Taft, distinguished lawyer, once said, "The listening ear implies humility, for it assumes a readiness to accept upsetting new ideas. The listening ear in which I believe also implies an eagerness for participation of others, both in discussion and in action."[7]

These two attributes—the ear that listens with humility, and the eagerness that welcomes the participation of others—are the most essential motivators of human beings. Listening also requires the sense of courage necessary to listen totally to another person's ideas, while at the same time we expose ourselves to the possibility of having some of our own ideas questioned. In listening with open ears, we temporarily put aside our own selfish needs and tend to give our attention and energies to being sympathetic and understanding of another's point of view.

Listening thus means not only *feeling for others* but implies an earnest attempt to commune or *experience with them.* As the famous semanticist, S. I. Hayakawa has said, "Listening requires entering actively and imaginatively into the other fellow's situation and trying to understand a frame of reference different from your own. This is not always an easy task."[8]

References

1. Wendell Johnson: *Your Most Enchanted Listener*. New York, Harper & Brothers, 1956, p. 60.
2. Harriet Van Horne: "'Martian Invasion' Night Revived," Column, *New York World-Telegram & Sun*, Oct. 1957.
3. Robert T. Oliver: *The Psychology of Persuasive Speech*. Longmans, Green and Co., 2nd Ed., 1957, p. 7, 367.
4. Wendell Johnson: "Do You Know How to Listen?" *E.T.C.*, xii, Autumn 1949.
5. Joost A. M. Meerloo: *Conversation and Communication*. New York, International Universities Press, Inc., 1952, p. 180.
6. *Ibid.*, p. 145.
7. Edward R. Murrow: *This I Believe*. New York, Simon and Schuster, 1952, p. 177.
8. S. I. Hayakawa: "How to Attend a Conference." *E.T.C.*, xiii, Autumn 1955, pp. 5-9.

The Magic of Listening

The magic of the tongue is the most dangerous of all spells.
—EDWARD BULWER LYTTON

EMERSON once said that "speech is power to persuade, to convert, to compel." Who of us, for instance, has not been swayed or influenced by the magic of religious ceremonies, parades, cheering sections, fraternity and club initiation rites. Word magic is present too in many of our colloquialisms, in our verbal directives and in the vernacular we use in predicting future events, while the verbalization of mystic refrains and the utterances of magic formulas of the *abracadabra, sesame, hocus pocus* variety are all thought in one way or another to possess miracle-working qualities on those areas over which they have influence.

The early philosophers regarded words as having power in themselves. To classify, they believed, was to name, and the name of a thing was its soul, its essence. Therefore to know the "name" word was to have power over mind and soul. This sorcery, known as the doctrine of the "Logos," is echoed in the beginning of the Gospel of St. John: "In the beginning was the *Word*, and the Word was with God, and the Word *was* God."

It would be difficult to erase the formidable imprints left upon us throughout history by the use of words. In every culture there have been priests, medicine-men, witch-doctors, shamans, exorcists or mediums said to be inspired with the magic of "gifted tongues" and alleged to communicate with the supernatural. The force and

65

magnitude of communicative language is vividly exemplified in the hieroglyphics of the Egyptians and in the Gospels of the *New Testament* with their word-of-mouth teachings of Jesus to His disciples. In conveying to the people the commandments of Jehovan, the Hebrew prophets used a direct: "Thus saith the Lord." So powerful was the authority of the prophets among the Hebrew people that the kings not infrequently trembled at their voices; for they were the direct instruments for the words of their God.

There are no people however primitive who are not affected by the magic of listening. It is said that one origin of words was in the imitation of sound—a "magic" attempt to master the sound-making object. In primitive times repetition and rhyming were long thought to be effective strategies against the threat of other sounds and words. Sounds and the din of chatter were first used to keep the evil spirits away. Many of us will still hum and whistle when we are afraid and alone in the dark.

According to Bronislaw Malinowski, "the main principle of magic belief is that words exercise power in virtue of their primeval mysterious connection with some aspect of reality . . . and the authority of spell-words is thought to have originated side by side "with animals and plants, with winds and waves, with human disease, human courage and frailty."[1]

However the concept in the language of *magic* arises not because words are thought to be conventional symbols of non-verbal facts, but because we who are listeners believe the word to be capable of casting a spell on an actual object and therefore of having power in itself. One might almost define such words as the *seeds* of word magic in which *the name gives power over the person or thing it signifies*.

In verbal magic we find implicit the belief that the statement or the utterance heard is enough to influence

66

situations. The person, the thing or the word which possesses the magic power is in itself able by its mere expression to produce the effect of magic and of the supernatural. For instance, the word "lizard" and the actual creature are felt to be *one and the same thing* because they arouse in us the same reactions. Levy-Bruhl explains in his book, *How Natives Think*, how primitive logic words on such a principle: the creature frightens us; the word when listened to frightens us; i.e.—the creature and the word are felt as being one and the same, thereby establishing a "mystic connection between the two."

Magic was once used among the Trobianders in their primitive ceremonies designed to bring about the growth of plants. An accredited magician having received a sequence of words, i.e., a spell, would then use it in well-organized ritualistic fashion.

> During the numerous rites of growth magic the voice is made to sweep the soil of each plot and thus to reach the tubers underground, the growing vine and its developing foliage. . . . In every act the magician's breath is regarded as the medium by which the magical force is carried. The voice—and let us remember it must be the voice of the accredited and fully instructed magician, and that his voice must correctly utter the words of an absolutely authentic spell—"generates" the power of the magic. This force is either directly launched on the earth or the tuber or the growing plant, or else it is indirectly conveyed by the impregnation of a substance, usually herbs, which is then applied to the object to be affected: the earth, the saplings, the *kamkokola* or the harvested taro or yams.[2]

In this example, as Malinowski points out, there is a definite connection between the word and the implied magical meanings which we as people give to them during the process of listening.

In the study of the texts and formulas of primitive

magic, it was found that there are three typical elements associated with the belief in magical efficiency.[3] There are, first, the phonetic effects or imitations of natural sounds such as the whistling of the wind, the growling of thunder, the roar of the sea, the voices of various animals. These sounds, because they symbolize certain phenomena, are believed either to produce them magically, or to express certain emotional states associated with the desire to be realized by means of the magic.

The second element, commonly used in primitive spells, is the use of words which invoke, state, or command the desired aim. Thus a sorcerer to make himself effective will mention all the symptoms of the disease which he is inflicting, or in a lethal formula he will describe the end of his victim. In *healing* magic, "the wizard will give word pictures of perfect health and bodily strength." In *economic* magic, "the growing of plants, the approach of animals, the arrival of fish in shoals are depicted." Again the magician in influencing his audience will "use words and sentences which express the motion under the stress of which he words his magic, and the action which gives expression to his emotion." The sorcerer will also increase the tone of his voice to a state of fury and will repeat such words as "I break," "I twist," "I burn," "I destroy," associating each with various parts of the body or internal organs of his subject. In such performances, the spells are based upon the same pattern as the rites and the words are selected as the substance of magic.

Finally, there is a third element in almost every spell for which there is no counterpart in ritual—the "mythological allusions, the references to ancestors and cultural heroes from which this magic has been received."

Words and sounds have a hypnotic and mystic effect upon our ears. In certain psychic phenomena such as those grouped under the heading of *telekinesis*, we find included movements of objects which are caused by the presence of a *medium* rather than through any force known to normal science. Tables tilt and are elevated, objects are thrown about, tambourines are rung. Another set of phenomena includes clairvoyance and clairaudience. In all of these the observer is *dependent solely upon the word of the medium who sees and hears things unseen or unheard by the observer*. In more complex manifestations the medium goes into a trance-like state and then talks, often using different voices which ramble on disconnectedly, give advice, answer questions the while professing to be voices of deceased persons who deliver messages from the spirit world. Some mediums supposedly have revealed secrets not known to any living person but their hearers and their "controls." This they accomplished by the use of such intimate names, memories, or personal turns of thought and speech that they frequently satisfied those present that they were in contact with the spirits of deceased friends and relatives. The talking medium is, however, only one method through which communication with the spirits and ghosts is made.

The development of mediumship often begins with rappings and the movement of articles of furniture. Next the rappings are codified—some signifying yes, others, no. Usually there is the forming and spelling out of words by means of an alphabet of raps. As the seance continues, the impatience of controls and mediums to speed up the process leads to use of the spoken word. Sometimes the communications are made by writing in which the experimenter thinks of something and his hand writes automatically. A host of experiments carried out in the 1800's by France's Pierre Felix Janet and others show that, far from being evidence of communication with a spirit world, these were but the normal channels for the outpourings of the operator's own subconscious mind.

The alluring influence of phonetics on the listening ear is further exemplified by the natives of the Trobriand

69

Islands. It is said that late in November as the rainy weather sets in, the natives find little work to do on the land. The fishing season is not yet in full swing and sociability is in the air. The festive mood lingers on after the traditional harvest dancing and feasting; and time is heavy on their hands as the bad weather keeps them at home. On a typical lazy evening, the natives congregate around a fireplace to talk. Sooner or later someone will be asked to tell a story, for this is the season of *fairy tales*. If he recites well, he soon provokes aliveness and laughter; others will join in, and in time this will develop into a regular performance.

Folk tales of a special type called *kubwonebu* are regularly recited in the villages. It is believed that these recitals have a beneficial influence on the new plants recently planted in the gardens. In order for this magic to be effective, a short ditty which alludes to a species of fertile wild plants known as *kasiyena* must always be recited at the end. Every story is "owned" by a member of the community, and though familiar to many, may be recited only by the "owner" who may, however, both teach it to another member of the tribe and authorize him to retell it. However, the art in telling an effective story is in knowing how to thrill and how to provoke hearty laughter, the main goals of any good teller of tales. A good raconteur knows just "how to change his voice in the dialogue, chant the ditties with due temperament, gesticulate, and in general play the gallery."[1]

> The following is an example of such a story: Two women go out in search of birds' eggs. One discovers a nest under a tree; the other warns her: "These are eggs of a snake, don't touch them." "Oh, no! They are eggs of a bird," says the first woman and carries them away. Some time later the mother snake comes back and finding the nest empty starts in search of the eggs. She enters the nearest village and sings a ditty:—

"I wend my way as I wriggle along,
The eggs of a bird it is licit to eat;
The eggs of a friend are forbidden to touch."

The search continues for a long time as the snake goes from one village to another and everywhere she sings her ditty. At last she reaches the village of the women and seeing the "culprit roasting the eggs, coils around her, and enters her body. The victim is laid down helpless and ailing. But the hero is nigh; a man from a neighboring village dreams of the dramatic situation, arrives on the spot, pulls out the snake, cuts it to pieces, and marries both women, thus carrying off a double prize for his prowess."[3]

In all of these stories, the text is extremely important. Without the context they would remain lifeless. However the impact of the effect on the native's ear is dependent wholly on the nature of the performance—the voice and the mimicry of the narrator, and his power to stimulate and make his audience respond. To be effective the performance is usually set for a particular hour of the day when the magic of the fairy tales has its greatest impact.

The Child's Use of Magic

The term "magic gesture" was first used by Ferenczi to describe one aspect of a baby's attempt to grasp reality via omnipotence. It represents the third of the infant's four stages in acquiring a sense of reality. This is the stage in which the child gives signs—in sucking movements of his mouth, the stretching of his hands toward objects, etc.—and misconceives the response of his environment as the result of his own omnipotence.

Words and magic were once one and the same thing and today words still retain much of their magic power. The achievement of the faculty of speech is experienced by a child as the acquisition of a great power which turns the "omnipotence of thought" into the "omnipotence of words." Consequently his earliest use of words is a charm directed toward influencing and forcing the external world to do those things that have been conjured up in words. He learns both to use and listen with respect to the omnipotence of words. His speech, so he discovers, becomes an instrument for the mastery and manipulation of his environment. He further discovers that if he can persuade and influence others to listen to him and be at his command, he will invariably receive affection and reassurance.

Early in his development, the child begins to recognize the importance of having his parents pay attention and listen to him. His mother becomes the more patient and sympathetic listener and so she is experienced as a "magic helper." He begins to recognize the mastery and power of his magic gestures and how to use these effectively—until the day when reality itself proves him wrong.

As the child grows and develops, he is even more dependent upon the magic of words. Although his intellectual processes are concrete and even animistic, the six-year-old is susceptible to semi-abstract symbols, charms and conjurations. He is greatly influenced by adult authority. For example, witness the modern version of primitive magic wherein the incantatory parent counts 1-2-3-4-5-6- with the understanding that when the magic 7 is uttered the agreed upon action will be carried through by the obedient child. In most cases the magic works. This procedure is based on pure suggestion and gullibility. The deliberate counting may be shortened or lengthened to suit the child's needs, thus giving him a support and an opportunity to mobilize enough energies of his own to make the proper adjustment.

The six-year-old, according to Gesell and Ilg, vascillates between two choices, the "good" and the "bad" in himself and his acts. He fears being rejected, and this leads him to search for constant approbation from his mother or to look to his "magic helper" in the control of his naughtiness. "Badness" separates him emotionally from his mother and this he wants to prevent at all costs. As he sees it, he can do nothing "bad or wrong" as long as he listens to and obeys her. For what purpose parents if not to determine allowed and forbidden things?

At the age of six, a child's interest in magic is strong. He plays that he is magic, has magic ears, uses counting as a magical maneuver, and adheres firmly to his sense of omnipotence. By the time he is eight, his belief in magic diminishes and his interests in this area become more objective. He does not believe as much in his omnipotent structure, is more aware of his surroundings, and is able to verbalize ideas and problems. He is also becoming less self-centered, uses his ears to listen more objectively. His listening as a whole becomes less magical and more realistic in nature. By the time he is ten years old, he has an increasingly realistic conception of the world, does not resort as much to fairy tales. He begins to emerge as an independent and critical thinker whose language and hearing are used as tools of communication. His radio and reading interests increase, listening becomes highly selective, and he acquires an extended use of code language.

The child now employs words as a part of his strategy of control, believing that through expression of the suitable word he can gain power over the object it represents. Children believe that magically they can change the external world with words in the same that psychotics do with their self-coined words. Every creator, as Meerloo states, "has a feeling of power over what he depicts; he feels himself to be magician and sorcerer. Infantile thoughts always contain this element of magic control of reality, for the infant is not yet capable of abstraction."[4] The child thinks that, by knowing the name of the object to which he refers, he can control, understand or manipulate it to suit his own needs. By verbalizing the name he can act on the thing, and, similarly, by changing the name he can change the thing. The thing then, to his way of thinking, *is* its name. The concept of the name as an abstraction comes much later.

As the child matures, he accepts to a continually greater degree the omnipotence of words and thoughts. To listen to or to speak the right or the wrong words comes to have significant importance. He learns, as do primitives, that he too can resort to the strategy of commanding his world with symbolic actions and words. He learns that words are powerful and destructive and should be used with care and discretion. Each word uttered may carry a "life or death significance."

The Logic of Superstition

Magic beliefs and practices originated not out of thin air but because of man's inner need to feel protected or secure against imagined threats to himself. These were the result of feared experiences actually lived through in which man received by chance a revelation of his power to attain the desired end and to communicate these same experiences to others.

Superstition is, in essence, a surviving trend—or hangover—of ways of thinking belonging to earlier stages of human development. As Jastrow says, "Superstition is crude, primitive, ignorant, dominated by fear and wish; it belongs historically and logically in a world in which magic, not science, prevails, in which things happen in ways mysterious and little understood."[5]

Men were never content merely to observe signs, to read omens of good or ill luck. They had to go on to invent various devices and forces for control. Thus charms, amulets and the complicated systems of witchcraft came into being. For example, in wishing the death of your enemy, you could, if you lived in days of yore, "make an image of his person, secure a lock of his hair, or the parings of his fingernails, or a piece of his clothing, and then stick thorns into it, burn it, torture it, bury it—all in the expectation that these injuries would befall your enemy."[5] This then was your magical procedure.

Natural forces personified became gods, rulers of earth and sea and sky, dispensers of human fate in superhuman fashion. Men regarded them with fear and religious awe, their ill will to be avoided, their good will sought, their intentions ascertained. To communicate with these forces and to invoke them necessitated a special art and out of that need developed the go-between or priestly medium who was a magician or sorcerer. He had the unique ability in the use of charms and secret controls and his magic powers for exercising these forces at will on whomsoever he wished. We all have heard of the influence of the medicine man in certain primitive tribes and of his power to remove an "evil eye" or break a spell cast upon an ill-fated man.

The language of superstition implies very little logic or reason, yet we have used it for centuries. Consider some of the following popular survivals: when you have not been affected by illness over a period of time, you rap on wood; when you sneeze, someone says "God bless you," or "Gesundheit!" You cross your fingers before an examination or a competitive attempt, or before asking for a raise. If you accidentally walk under a ladder, you cautiously and anxiously retrace your steps backward. If you spill salt, you toss a pinch over your left shoulder; or, if you don't want to hear about some dire probable happening, you say peremptorily, "Don't say it—you'll make it happen!"

The notion that words have power over realities and life-facts is a negative concept of language. By automatically conforming to, and listening to, and believing that there is some mystical power in language, we find ourselves confronted with problems of misevaluation.

75

Words in themselves are not unique but only refer to objects, situations and feelings as such. They do not contain inherent magical or invested powers of authority. Man himself, because of his cultural habits and his mode of listening, has introduced this system of misevaluated interpretation. The following illustrates the evil power given certain words in distant places:

> The natives of Madagascar are reluctant to speak of lightning; the Baziba never mention earthquakes; rain is not mentioned by name in Samoa; fire is not named in China where there is a risk of conflagration; the ancient Scandinavians also observed the same precaution, and they did not use the ordinary word for water while making beer, lest the brew should turn out flat.[6]

Social Taboos on Words

The correct or proper word or the soothing expression attracts and charms listeners. In contradistinction, vulgar, dirty or expressive words are to be avoided at all cost.

We have a tendency in our culture to feel that certain words have different musical effects, while others are too "ugly" or "strong" for our ears. We place affective connotations on certain specific words which in turn act as verbal taboos and provide obstacles in communication. For instance, we make all sorts of attempts magically to change and to replace the evil, the undesirable, the negative, the dangerous expression, by "good" words so that what we say will make the content more acceptable in itself as well as to our listeners or readers.

A euphemism is the substitution of inoffensive or mild expression for a word or phrase that may offend or suggest something unpleasant. Their use in a substitution is one way in which we attempt to protect ourselves from the painful aspects of reality. By closing our ears to anything unpleasant by changing it into softer, more acceptable terms—a magical maneuver widely used in our society—

we manage to allay and subdue the tone of sounds or words having strong affective connotations. Some of our verbal taboos, especially religious ones, originate in our belief that the names of gods are too holy to be heard or spoken. However not all verbal taboos can be explained by word-magic. According to some psychologists, our reluctance to discuss certain areas of sex and bodily functions is due to the fact that we all have certain areas of inhibition which are so distasteful that we do not like to admit their presence even to ourselves. Because we fear having our illusions of being right and proper disturbed, we try not to listen to words which remind us of these.

In the Victorian era—and almost as much today—words having to do with sex had a strong resistance value. We have a tendency to change the subjective meaning of obscene words or other affective terms by the particular context or emotional coloring we give to them at the time of listening. For instance, for some reason we feel it socially permissible to use certain expressive "dirty" words when we are with friends or acquaintances; yet when we are with others, the use of the same words will have a prohibitive connotation. In place of a simple word like *toilet*, we use such terms as *rest room, lavatory, lounge*, "*He*" or "*She*" *rooms*. We also use formal anatomical terms, such as *intercourse, penis, vagina, defecate, urinate*, in place of certain simpler and more expressive terms which most of us know but reject because of a kind of public censorship and the numerous and complicated verbal taboos placed upon us in our society.

Social-wise it is also more polite and soothing to the ear to say *expectorate* instead of *spit*, *inebriation* rather than *drunkenness*, to *pass away* or *depart* rather than to *die*, *retire* than *go to bed*. Most of us use these verbal stratagems not merely to give different names to things, but because these words when spoken have strong affective connotations too painful to the average ear.

Aside from words with sexual meaning, we find words with strong affective connotations in many social areas—racial, national, religious and political. For example, the word *red* or *communist* immediately registers in many of our ears a feeling of antagonism and contempt and may even suggest that the person so labeled should be jailed, punished or prosecuted. In still others who have strong prejudices and fear admitting these prejudices to themselves, the substitution of makeshift words gives them a protective wall behind which they can hide their real feelings.

In our mass-conscious radio, television and movie industries, there is a serious concern about avoiding words which might prove embarrassing or forbidden to the ear drum. Any form of profanity, obscenity or blasphemy is considered reprehensible and as such its utterance is forbidden. Words like "bowels," "damn," "hell," "God," "Lord," "Jesus," "Christ"—unless used reverently, "broad" as applied to a woman, and many other such similar so-called prohibitive terms are condemned. All of these are words we all know and use in our everyday conversations, yet they would shock and embarrass us should they be mentioned in these mass media.

In short, the use of magic in language produces destructive and adverse consequences to our personalities as a whole and leads to a distortion of life-facts. It also places the burden of emphasis in communication on irrational premises and not actualities. If we would listen effectively, it is essential that we evaluate our words in their true context and not give to them supernatural magic powers. Man must ultimately discard the habit of assuming that language has in it sacrosanct or tabooed ingredients. Words have no authority in themselves or magical equivalents. It is up to us as listeners, as effectors of communication, to discard the out-moded magical rituals in language and to think of words as no more than symbols of factual representation. To do otherwise is a step toward confusion, misevaluation and a reverting back to the primitive and the infantile.

References

1. Bronislaw Malinowski: *Magic, Science and Religion.* New York, Doubleday Anchor Book, 1954.
2, 3. Bronislaw Malinowski: *Ibid.*, p. 103.
4. Joost A. M. Meerloo: *Conversation and Communication.* New York, International Universities Press, 1952, p. 72.
5. Joseph Jastrow: *Effective Thinking.* New York, The World Publishing Company, 1931, pp. 149-152.
6. Robert Briffault: *The Mothers.* New York, Macmillan Company, 1927, I, p. 15.

Listening to the Essence of things

He who has ears to hear, let him hear.
—St. Mark

W HEN we listen totally and with meaningful purpose we listen to the essence of things. There is an art to listening. *To listen fully* we should be in an open and receptive state of mind, for only when we are in an "accepting" mood is our full attention given. *To listen effectively* we should abandon and put aside all prejudices, preconceived judgments, taboos and other activities.

Psychologically, the concept *listening* indicates a definite and usually voluntary effort to comprehend acoustically. This differs greatly from the more inclusive concept of hearing which is the mere reception of stimuli over auditory pathways. *Successful* listening presupposes hearing and *precedes* understanding.

We must further differentiate between active *holistic* listening and passive *vicarious* listening. In listening actively, the individual does so with *all* of his self—his senses, his attitudes, beliefs, thoughts and intuitions. In passive listening, the listener becomes an organ for the reception of sound and has little self-perception, personal involvement, "gestalt" discrimination, or even live curiosity.

The good listener is constantly aware of himself and of how he can give more of himself to the exchange. He works with his ears, his eyes, his whole being. It takes a deal of energy to listen productively and at the same time to remain actively involved and yet be keenly curious. Effective listening cannot be accomplished simply by remaining passive and allowing the words to pour into our ears. It involves the tapping and drawing upon our senses as receptors and a transmitting back to us of information which can be assimilated and made available for future use.

To listen well, one must have the capacity and the desire to examine critically, to evaluate and reshape values, attitudes and relationships to oneself and to others. In so doing, one must learn to listen with "open ears" and to be patient with oneself.

Before communication can be meaningful, the speaker, the listener and the thing or situation discussed must have some mutual relationship. Both speaker and listener must define their terms and know what they are attempting to understand. Otherwise the essential purpose of their meeting is defeated. There should be levels of agreement not only on the facts but on the whole basic content. Thus both speaker and listener must assume equal responsibility for their part in the total situation, have mutual respect for each other and be wholeheartedly open to each other's criticism and opinions.

The way in which we listen can change the meaning and context of our daily living. The healthy listener, for instance, differs from the disturbed listener in that he reacts to most situations with an inner feeling of strength and freedom, security and self-confidence. He does not feel compelled to listen to everything that is said or that is silently implied. He is free to choose that which has meaning for him personally while at the same time he is able to relate it to the total situation. And once he makes his decision and voluntary selection, he will accept responsibility for his choice.

One cannot be too egocentric or prejudiced. The listener who is tense and anxious is one who fears mutual exchange of ideas. He is constantly in doubt and suspicious about the actions and motives of others and therefore his listening becomes highly attuned to criticism and rebuff, making him hypersensitive, cautious, defensive and constantly on his guard. Since man's very existence depends upon his ability to exchange information and to remain in communication with his fellow man, listening which does not further these aims can only be disturbing.

Every person who makes a statement desires to be understood and accepted. If he can evoke an understanding and an accepting response from his listener, he derives pleasure and satisfaction. Appropriate response is therefore important for psychological growth. On the other hand, an inappropriate reply or improper timing of listening responses is often taken as an indication of disapproval or rejection.

To be listened to with patience and understanding, to reach a quick and mutual agreement, and to be understood, is a pleasure. It is what we all strive for, and if such gratification is experienced over and over again, an individual or group is likely to be well informed, adaptable and capable of withstanding frustration.

In any discussion, for example, we find a speaker, A, who is attempting to express an idea or put something across, and a listener, B, who is endeavoring to grasp what is being said in its true context. Theoretically speaking, therefore, successful communication takes place when both parties involved reach corresponding levels of agreement as to the established information.

In practice, however, as Ruesch[1] has stated in his *Disturbed Communication*, nobody can prove that such a state has been achieved. We can only infer from certain indices derived from the communicative behavior of the participants whether agreement has been reached. The most significant criterion of agreement is found in the acknowledgment of A's statement by B and the effect such acknowledgment has upon A. In the process of communication, Ruesch offers four possibilities that must be distinguished. Briefly summarized they are:—

1. *Acknowledgment* of receipt of statement with *understanding:* In the actual exchange, two sections are being considered: A's attempts to get an idea across and B's endeavor to listen to and *understand* what A is trying to say.

   When B fully acknowledges A's statements in terms which are qualitatively and quantitatively satisfactory to A, he indeed expresses in word, gesture or action the following: I fully understand; I appreciate what you say; I get it.

   Such positive acknowledgment indicates that a level of agreement has been reached by B who in turn signals to A that he believes that correspondence of information has been established. When A perceives this acknowledgment, he relates this to himself and to the whole situation. If B's acknowledgment matches A's expectations and A signals to B that such is the case, mutuality of understanding has occurred. A's experience of being understood is related to his ability to elicit in B a piece of information similar to the one held by himself. The success of this mutual exchange between speaker and listener produces a sensation of pleasure.

2. *Acknowledgment* of receipt of statement *without understanding:* When A makes a statement, he anticipates several possibilities: first, that he will be understood; second, that he will not be understood; third, that his statement will be distorted. As he assesses these possibilities, he attempts to determine whether or not B as he listens is disposed to perceive his intentions. Regardless of whether B does or does not understand A's statement, B's readiness to explore A's intentions, his interest in listening to what A has to say and his curiosity to grasp the way A feels is reflected in an easily perceived attitude. This indication of readiness to understand is equated with acceptance and is

gratifying, irrespective of whether or not understanding can be achieved or agreement can be reached. Therefore, *negative* acknowledgment, implying immediate lack of understanding but readiness to listen further, can be as gratifying as *positive* acknowledgment that the statement has been understood. In this latter case, B may express in word, gesture or action one of the following: I do not understand; I do not get it; say it differently; elaborate further.

3. *Acknowledgment* of *mutual agreement:* Acknowledgment of agreement existing between A and B in terms which are qualitatively and quantitatively satisfactory to both involves such reciprocal statements as: we got together; we made a deal; I am of the same opinion as you are; we have the same interests.

Levels of agreement are never absolute or complete. They vary from individual to individual and from situation to situation. Agreements are also limited in time and as to subject matter. If they were complete, man's chances for survival would be reduced by elimination of alternative ways of thinking and acting.

The pleasure experienced in reaching an agreement is somewhat different from the pleasure experienced in being understood. Understanding requires sympathy and the benevolent attitude of another person, while agreement is more closely allied to the facts of the situation. Thus it is easier to reach a limited agreement than it is to be fully understood. Agreements can be reached without true understanding, but if agreement is accompanied by complete mutual understanding, then the pleasure experienced is extremely gratifying.

4. *Acknowledgment* of *mutual disagreement:* Understanding and nonunderstanding, agreement and disagreement occur in the process of healthy, normal and potentially successful communication. But if misunderstanding and disagreement become goals in themselves, then we deal with a pathological process of communication.

Acknowledgment is a particular form of response. It involves recognition of the fact that a statement has content. It is often exaggerated by those who "lay it on thick" and by persons who dramatize. Such response on the part of a listener is disconcerting to the average speaker whom it overstimulates, frustrates and often embarrasses. In contrast, poorly timed acknowledgment cuts the pleasure of control and often prevents completion of a communication. Listeners of this sort, knowing that human beings crave acknowledgment, will withhold their immediate responses as a means of frustrating and tormenting others.

Qualitatively deviant acknowledgement of a statement on the part of the listener also provokes displeasure and frustration. This response in many instances is extremely a statement, the receiver disregards the sender's intent. This Ruesch has called the *tangential reply* and he has cited the following example as illustration:

> Johnny comes running toward his mother joyously shouting, "Look, I caught a worm!" Mother looks at Johnny and in a dry-, pleasure-killing voice remarks, "Go and wash your dirty hands." The child, entirely deflated, disappointed, and confused, enters the house. By directly initiating a new message—the order to wash hands—when she saw the mud-covered fingers of her youngster, she in fact disregarded his intentional statement. Had the mother said, "Yes, this is a lovely worm," and paused, she then could have initiated a new message, "and now you go and wash your dirty hands."[2]

In administering a tangential reply, the receiver or listener takes cognizance of the sender's intention to communicate but disregards the content of his statement. By responding with a side remark, he tends to confuse the sender who may not understand the connection between statement and reply. Therefore, in replying tangentially, the listener deprives the speaker of the pleasure of being understood and at the same time, the receiver

85

attempts to throw his sender off guard by making another statement to which the receiver also expects an acknowledgment.

This form of verbal strategy is used by conversational sharks who attempt to demonstrate their superiority in the speaking situation. They base their alleged strength on the fact that others will, from a weakened position, take the trouble to reply to the new topic introduced; they assume that these others will not reply in a tangential way. This can be particularly devastating when the affected person is unaware of the shift that has taken place. This is what is commonly referred to as "making a monkey" out of the other individual. If in a conversation both speaker and listener engage in tangential replies, the exchange becomes disconnected and eventually breaks down and communication becomes disturbed as both participants struggle to understand each other and to reach further levels of agreement.

The Importance of Selectivity in Listening

In effective listening, it is essential that we know we cannot perceive everything as it is or appears to be. As human beings we can only see and listen to the fullest extent of our individual capacities, feelings, beliefs and potentialities, knowing that in every situation some degree of total comprehension and finer detail will be blotted out of the total picture.

The human mind is so adapted that it attempts to treat successively that which in nature happens simultaneously. Similarly in everyday situations a listener cannot at once respond to all the shadings of another person's statements. Although the listener tries to be selective in replying first to one part and then to another, in reality he rarely gets around so doing because in the meantime new topics of interest will have arisen. Thus, in replying, the listener will select his responses to fit certain aspects or parts of the message and discard such others as he thinks irrelevant. His acknowledgment in its final form will be an interpretative response to the statement of the speaker or it will become a new message to which he expects the other person to reply.

The effects of poor selectivity in listening are a major source of disturbance in child-parent relationships. Parents greatly influence their children who in turn look up to and imitate them and a parent who provides his child with little or no selectivity of action greatly hinders the child's psychological growth.

The most powerful tool in producing defective evaluation then is the *tangential response*. This most frequent form of interference both provides a child with the elements of choice and prejudices the outcome. For example, the parent asks, "Which of these guns would you like?" The child makes his choice and is told that the selected gun is too expensive. The frustrated child is then made to accept the gun his parent had chosen in the first place. Had the parent said at the beginning "This is the only one we can afford," the tangential response could have been avoided. When the child is exposed repeatedly to influences of this sort, his listening becomes defective. He cannot learn to weigh information in its totality but will tend to let one factor prejudice the outcome.

Effective listening should be encouraged in the early developmental years by the permitting of situations where there is multiple choice. However disturbances will result when parents teach their children to reduce the number of possibilities to two. Even in adulthood this narrowing of choice-possibility compels one to listen in terms of fixed limits which will disturb a proper evaluation of the whole picture.

Another most important factor in selective listening is the ability to choose and grasp that quantity of information which can be both stimulating and yet produce effective movement in the total communicative experience.

In order for the listener to achieve this optimal state of concentration, he must be alert and attentive. He must be in a relaxed receptive mood, able to focus his whole body in the direction of the speaker. "The listener, writes Oliver, "leans toward it, his muscles taut, his eyes intent, his ears strained, his very breathing stopped . . ."[3]

At such a time the whole body becomes vibrant and alive, latent powers rise to the surface and are brought to bear upon the solution of the task. The hearing sense becomes keener than it normally is. Other sounds that ordinarily predominate slowly fade into the background of consciousness or disappear entirely. The mind reaches forward as it becomes more acutely aware of the object of its attention. Ultimately, as clarity, understanding and true perception are reached, this concentration of attention fosters the solution of problems that will otherwise seem too difficult to attempt.

To reach a high level of attentive listening, the body must be tense, ready, expecting—the converse of "relaxed and indifferent." In attentive listening, the mind attends to a stimuli, seeks for it, examines it, evaluates it, and selects from it that which can prove both stimulating and activating. Other bodily processes take a secondary role and temporarily slow down or stop as the individual makes an all out effort to encompass the object of his attention.

Attentiveness in listening runs hand in hand with aliveness in interest. The two terms are inseparably intertwined. However even under the most favorable circumstances, the attention may sometimes wander. As human beings, *our limit of absolute attention is only a few seconds.* We like variety and are easily distracted, swayed, grow restless or indifferent. When we do not listen with real attention or interest, the information at hand seems monotonous and boring. This leads to disturbed listening.

In testing the number of objects that can be taken in in a single perception, psychologists expose them for only one-fifth of a second. At longer intervals, the observer may shift his attention. In like fashion the attention of most listeners demands variety. In addition to demanding variety for our attention, we suffer from such realistic inhibiting factors as fatigue, drowsiness, emotional blocks or environmental distractions. To overcome these distractions and counterattractions, we must exert extra effort toward healthy listening. To sit back and demand to be passively stimulated limits our true capacity for listening. In listening with purpose, we must inject ourselves into the situation, and we must be open and receptive enough to give our fullest energies to whatever we are listening to so as to produce an effect of both acknowledgment and understanding. Only in so doing can real communication be achieved.

In everyday living, *selective* listening is most important. Too many of us listen to radio, television and recordings with too little self-discrimination. We expose ourselves aurally to all sorts of noises in an automaton-like manner, rarely questioning the "why" or "what" of what we are hearing. Selective listening is the opposite of turning on the radio or television set and letting any sort of noise blare forth. It requires self-evaluation and a choice or choices as to what may be of value. With such active participation, we project ourselves with more aliveness into the situation and so will derive real profit and pleasure from our listening.

Selectivity in listening is essential whether listening to friends, attending lectures or listening to a sermon in church. In these and other verbal situations, the listener can develop a good rapport with the speaker and thus absorb a great deal of information, or he can leave empty handed and untouched. The listener derives from the actual experience only that which he gives to it, his pleasure and satisfaction growing in proportion to his degree of involvement.

We think much faster than we talk. The average rate of speech for most Americans to repeat, is around 125 words per minute. This rate is slow when we consider that the human brain is made up of more than thirteen billion cells capable of solving the most complicated problems. We human beings use but an infinitesimal part of the brain's functioning capacity. That this is so is in great measure due to our not knowing how to think or concentrate well and, indirectly, to our inability to listen effectively. In reading, however, we are able to measure more accurately how fast the brain can handle words. Some people can read and understand up to 1,200 words per minute; others by concentrated effort even more, possibly because there are fewer distractions in reading than in listening.

Studies in the speech field show that some people can understand words spoken at a faster rate than the average 125 per minute. It has been demonstrated that speech can be comprehended at more than 300 words per minute without significant loss over what can be taken in and retained at much slower speeds. Therefore, many more spoken words can be listened to and understood than it is possible to form words orally without mechanical distortion ending in unintelligibility.

Though the brain can deal with words at a lightning pace, we as humans have the capacity to be selective and to receive words realistically at a much slower pace. We can regulate the complex mechanism of hearing by slowing down our thinking and by adapting our listening to the 125-word-per-minute speech rate. However, this is a most difficult process when we continue to think at high speed while the spoken words enter at low speed. To quote from Nichols and Stevens, "the differential between thinking and speaking rates means that our brains work with hundreds of words in addition to those we hear, assembling thoughts other than those spoken to us. To put it another way, we can listen and still have spare time for thinking."[4] It is what you do with this spare thinking time that determines the quality of your listening and this, in turn, holds the key to effective listening.

Let us now try to understand how our brain helps us to store up memories for future use.

The Stream of Consciousness

The human brain is one of the most marvelous of all the marvels of living nature. It weighs but fifty ounces and occupies a volume of about 1,500 cubic centimeters or about one and one-half quarts. Yet despite its size and weight, it contains about ten billion cells grouped into geographical-like areas each subdivided into smaller areas, in which are hidden life's greatest mysteries and miracles. All of this encompasses one of the greatest of creations— the human mind.

For years scientists have been engaged in the study and mapping of the brain in an effort to localize its infinite functions in terms of human responses conscious, subconscious and unconscious, involuntary and voluntary. Much progress has been made in the last century in localizing the brain centers controlling such functions as sight, smell, hearing, touch and other sensory perceptions. Yet as William L. Laurence wrote in a *New York Times* article, "the human brain still remains a vast, unexplored 'no-man's-land,' the greatest mystery of them all, that of the mind itself, still eluding man's most intensive probings."[5]

At the annual meeting of the National Academy of Sciences, Dr. Wilder Penfield, Director of the Montreal Neurological Institute and one of the world's leading authorities on brain function, reported on a mechanism discovered in the brain which unlocks stream-of-consciousness records. By stimulating the brains of human subjects with tiny electrical currents, a new area was found which

91

gave most valuable information. It seems there is hidden away in this area of the brain a record of the stream-of-consciousness. This stream, laid down during man's waking or conscious hours, is a complete record of happenings which have occurred during his periods of conscious awareness—details one might hope to remember for a brief space only and which are later lost to voluntary recall.

Its content never the same from moment to moment; the record of this stream, brought to light by the stimulating electrodes, might be likened, according to Dr. Penfield, to the operation of a wire recorder or a continuous film strip with sound track. In describing an experiment, Dr. Penfield reported that when a certain region of the area was stimulated by the electrode, his patient heard a long forgotten song, not as though he were imagining the tune himself but was actually hearing it. However he did not know *why* he heard that particular song.

Other patients experimented upon by Dr. Penfield reported that experiences brought back by the electrode were much more real than remembering. And yet at the same time they were aware of the present. Still others cried out in astonishment that they were hearing and seeing friends they knew were far distant.

In his conclusions, Dr. Penfield has labeled this particular area in the temporal cortex "the area for comparative interpretation" or the "interpretive cortex." With its help, experiences which have been heard, seen or felt and stored somewhere in our subconscious minds can be unlocked and scanned for the purpose of automatic interpretation of the present, and with the aid of this invaluable mechanism we are able to make conscious comparisons of present experiences with similar past experiences.

In summary we may say that everything that is transmitted by sound wave is utilized by our hearing mechanism. If we are within earshot of a sound, our stream-of-consciousness has the capacity to retain even the most minute effects. Even though at times we may appear not to be paying direct attention or if we seem not to understand the words we hear, they are being recorded somewhere in our mental apparatus. Sometime later this absorption makes it possible for us to reproduce this same material without doing so intentionally. In essence, nothing passes through our ears that we do not hear and tuck away somewhere in the storage rooms of our unconscious.

Improving Our Listening Skills

Today little emphasis is placed on the art or skill of listening. For too long our listening training has taken the form of such admonitions as, "Pay attention!" or "Open up your ears!" or "Listen to this!"

Listening ability depends largely on intelligence. It is assumed that "bright" people are good listeners and that "dull" ones listen poorly. It is not uncommon to hear such phrases as "he doesn't listen to anything" or "he's stupid" or "you haven't heard a word I said."

There is no doubt that intelligence has much to do with our ability to listen. On the other hand we tend to exaggerate its importance. A poor listener need not necessarily be a stupid person. To be a good listener, one must apply certain skills that have to be learned either through experience or training. Without these listening skills, the ability to grasp what is heard will be low whether one is a person of high or low intelligence.

In a series of tests at the University of Minnesota, Nichols and Stevens concluded that although women had higher average intelligence scores on the listening tests, 95 out of 100 males were better listeners. In another series of tests in which the subjects were divided according to their parents' occupations, those who came from farm families turned out to be the best listeners. Yet these children were not the highest in intelligence tests given at the same time.

Listening ability is also not necessarily allied to hearing acuity. A person whose ears function properly is not for that reason better equipped to be a good listener. Statistics have shown that only six per cent or less of the nation's school children are troubled by hearing defects, yet difficulty in understanding what is heard is most prevalent. So we see that effective listening requires much more than just healthy ears or the ability to read well, that it is an art which requires serious training and practice over a period of years. Children will imitate their parents in either good or bad listening habits, but in later years, one learns to strengthen listening skills—or to weaken them—through the misuse of one's ears.

Effective listening is not a simple, passive act. It requires much concentration and mental effort. For instance, in listening to the radio or television, aural exposure is not enough. Selectivity of programs and active participation are essentials for careful listening. To profit and experience genuine listening pleasure, a certain degree of listening ability is necessary.

According to a study of high school students made recently in New York and New Jersey, the regular use of radio as a teaching aid stimulates student interest in and understanding of current events. This study included a home listening project followed by classroom discussion based on "The World at Large," a Columbia Broadcasting System public affairs radio series which covered high lights in the area of current history, with government officials, international political leaders and university faculty members participating.

Two groups of students were chosen for the home listening experiment. One group, assigned to listen to the five programs in the series, did so for a period of two weeks. The other or control group was not assigned to listen to the programs. At the end of the allotted time, teachers in the English and civics and social studies developed discussion units based on such material in the broadcasts as civil rights legislation, the World Health Organization, the Hungarian crisis, statehood for Alaska and Hawaii, and atomic energy.

The teachers who participated in the experiment agreed that students had learned more about current history by listening to public affairs presentations on the radio than by reading about them regularly in the newspaper. However, it was stressed that students did need guidance in selecting program material as the means for developing habits of purposeful rather than random listening.

In this same area, we have the spoken-word records. Libraries across the country have proven that good listening usually paves the way to reading and that one of the best ways to encourage a child to visit the library regularly and to enjoy what it has to offer is through storytelling hours.

The Curative Value of Listening

Effective listening can have a profound curative value. Most of us know the enjoyment and profit derived from listening to stimulating music, literature, poetry, drama or good conversation. Although listening in itself is not a cure-all for our basic problems, it can serve as a comforting agent in helping us to relax, to concentrate better, to become more aware of and move closer to our real selves.

To listen with purpose requires an inner strength and the courage to open our minds to other people's ideas, while at the same time we must face up to the fact that some of our own beliefs may be wrong. Lack of courage on the other hand results in a tenacity and stubborn resistance to change and an unwillingness to acknowledge defeat. It also prevents us from being flexible in most situations and from being sympathetic and opening our ears to whatever may be said.

The necessary attitude for a sympathetic and understanding listener cannot be learned or practiced. It must come from within, from the very human wish both to be heard and to listen to others. In order to *sound* sincere, one must *be* and *act* sincere. There must also be an empathy between speaker and listener, a feeling one for the other, and a deep sense of mutuality and respect.

The good listener must believe himself before he can expect belief from others. He must believe in the value of his own ideas and feelings and be honest with himself and others. He must also assume responsibility for his actions and admit to his own shortcomings. In so doing, he will listen with inner strength and conviction. Martin Block, who has made a most successful career of radio announcing, refuses to work for a sponsor whose product does not meet his own individual standards. Block's stand often fosters like convictions in his listener and so works to the advantage of his sponsors.

In conclusion, may I add that effective listening presupposes a certain state or feeling of "communicative empathy." It is the merging of one personality with another until some degree of identification is achieved. Given this identification or merger between speaker and listener, real understanding is possible. This identifying of one's self with the other person takes place to some extent in every conversation—it is the fundamental process in love and in human nature.

References

1. Jurgen Ruesch: *Disturbed Communication.* New York, Norton & Company, 1957, p. 37.
2. *Ibid.,* p. 54.
3. Robert T. Oliver: *The Psychology of Persuasive Speech.* New York, Longmans, Green and Co., 1957, 2nd ed., p. 118.
4. Ralph G. Nichols and Leonard A. Stevens: *Are You Listening?,* McGraw-Hill Book Company, Inc., 1957, p. 79.
5. William L. Laurence: "Science in Review." *New York Times,* Nov. 24, 1957.

The Disease of Not Listening

They have ears, but they hear not—

In the second part of *King Henry IV*, Lord Chief Justice says to Falstaff, "You hear not what I say to you," and Falstaff replies, "Very well, my Lord, very well; rather an't please you, it is the disease of not listening, the malady of not marking, that I am troubled withal."

Every person is equipped at birth with the apparatus which makes it possible for him to listen effectively and to communicate with others. Apart from the known organic disturbances of hearing, our listening patterns may be altered by the placing of our individual barriers in the way of good listening. We become involved in our own needs, narrow our scope of observation and become too deep in thought or distracted to pay attention to the messages of others.

Most of us do not know nor do we wish to learn how to listen. We go to lectures to hear what is talked about, yet we are not necessarily good listeners. Should the subject matter become a bit involved or require some extra thought on our part as listeners, our hearing becomes suddenly hazy and confusing, and the listening process is interfered with as distractions multiply. Even the speaker is lost in the shuffle.

For the last several years Ralph G. Nichols and Leonard A. Stevens, authors of the recent book *Are You Listening?*, have tested the ability of people to understand and remember what they hear. At the University of Minnesota

97

they examined the listening ability of several thousand students and of hundreds of business and professional people in adult-education courses. In each case the person tested listened to short talks by various faculty members and was then given a carefully constructed standard test designed to measure the subject's comprehension and retention of the aurally received material.

The general conclusion arrived at from these tests was that immediately after the average person has listened to someone else talk, he remembers only about half of what he heard—*no matter how carefully he thinks he has listened.*

It was further concluded by the investigators and confirmed by reports of research at Florida State University, Michigan State University and elsewhere that two months after listening to a person talk, the average listener will remember only about 25 per cent of what was said.

Paul T. Rankin, formerly Supervising Director of Research and Adjustment for the Detroit public schools, once made an interesting survey of the importance of better listening which attracted the attention of educators. He selected sixty-eight adults of different occupations and asked them to keep tabs every fifteen minutes of the amount of time they spent talking, reading, writing and listening. The survey was carried on by these people for approximately two months.

Rankin's results in this investigation point to the distressing need for better listening. He found that on the average his subjects spent seventy per cent of each waking day in verbal communication. He also learned that of this communicating time, the sixty-eight adults spent an average of nine per cent in writing, sixteen per cent in reading, thirty per cent in talking and forty-five per cent in listening.

The Rankin survey pointed up the need for more effective listening training that has been overlooked in our school systems from the very beginning. The eyes, as Nichols and Stevens state, "have occupied the favored position, with the visual skills of reading and writing getting chief attention. Meanwhile, the aural skills of speaking and listening have been kept in the background, improving in a hit-or-miss fashion, if at all."[1] The shortcomings of such an educational procedure become apparent when we leave school and find that personal communication most often depends upon the ear. The percentage of time spent in reading accordingly drops off rapidly while the need for listening perceptively increases.

The ear has long been the "neglected child" in our systems of communication. Yet listening is most important in the everyday communication of information. In business, for example, should people fail to hear and understand each other, the results are costly. Because of inefficient listening, millions of dollars are lost in industry each year. Industrial executives have come to realize the increasing importance of listening and its effect on business. Today this is considered so vital that industry is spending hundreds of millions of dollars to make its communicating systems work.

Social-wise the effects of poor listening can also be of a detrimental nature. In a recent *Look* article, "How American Teen-Agers Live," one of the major headings was: *Parents are "seen"—but not heard.* This article clearly and vividly describes the painful effects poor listening habits have on the youth of today. Teen-agers from coast to coast, finding it difficult to get their elders to listen to them, have created their own culture and rules of behavior. Frustrated in their attempts to win the help of parents and friends in guiding them through the most difficult years of their lives, they have been forced instead to find ways of entertaining themselves. Unable to communicate with the world about them, they have become victims of aloneness, with more "idle hours" than any other age group.

Too often the youth of today is bored, has little interest in himself or others, and so searches frantically for the means to fill his emptiness. He indulges compulsively in such activities as games, watching movies and TV, driving at a furious pace, dancing, eating and talking, always looking for a means of identification and self-acceptance, someone to listen to him, someone to understand him. All these his parents have denied him—these parents that are "seen" but not heard.

In their state of progressive discontent and frustration, these teen-agers resemble their parents in that they too do not listen effectively. It is not uncommon to hear parents complain that their children listen but don't hear them, yet a recent study by Gilbert Youth Research revealed that two-thirds of all teen-agers questioned said they had *listened* to the radio the previous day, three-fourths of them for *two hours or more* and mostly to rock 'n' roll!

There are more than 16,000,000 teen-agers in America, a statistic which points to the magnitude and importance of this problem. In addition to the confusions attendant upon our changing culture, external pressures and internal ferments, our most significant problem would seem to lie right in the home. The inability of parents to listen effectively and the associated scarcity of communication with their children is appalling. As the Youth Research reports, 76 per cent of our teen-agers "never discuss the facts of life with their parents."

Until parents assume more responsibility for the growth of their children, face the truth within themselves and listen more efficiently, the problem of teen-age deterioration will continue to exist. As someone has said, "better children can only come from better parents."

Origins of Faulty Listening

Basically the soil for healthy growth and productive listening must contain feelings of genuine warmth, love and respect. A child needs to feel that his environment is one in which he is wanted, loved, needed, one in which there is a sense of belonging. If these feelings are lacking, then an emotional stirring is generated which is difficult for the child to understand or accept and so he tends to become weak, insecure and shaky. This may easily become the focal point around which his uncertainty with its increasing frustrations and disappointments begins to be felt. Difficulties in listening can begin at this point.

Sometimes the parents, absorbed in their own problems, are incapable of giving adequate love or of listening with warmth and understanding, and this failure may be expressed either openly in the form of parental hostility toward an unwanted child or by the oversolicitude or self-sacrificing attitude of an "ideal mother." Should these parental threats begin at an early age, the child as a result of his emotionally weakened condition is unable to organize sufficient forces to restore order to his disorganized state. Instead he is pervaded with feelings of helplessness, isolation and hostility, the beginnings of basic anxiety. By way of achieving some form of safety and protection, the child may now be compelled to orient and direct his energies toward the adoption of a more modified way of life.

At first he does so by using *ad hoc* strategies—he conforms to his environment or withdraws from it as the situation dictates. Though such attempts are basically neurotic attempts to solve conflict, they do at first offer some means of aiming at a state of pseudo-unity and a lessening of inner chaos and turmoil. Ultimately however these same attitudes become invested with pride and so result in so-called virtues which only serve to reactivate the neurotic process.

The art of listening begins at home. Communication between parent and child should be, from birth on, a primary unifying force in the healthy development of the individual personality. The more solid and cohesive our emotional ties become at this time, the better equipped will we be to communicate with the outside world in later years.

Solidification of a family group depends to a large degree upon communication through the spoken word since man is essentially a speaking animal and makes himself best understood when he talks. The "talking" phase of family communication usually runs a natural course but the "listening" phase frequently gives rise to numerous problems. In a home which encourages freedom of thought and expression the members are free both to speak their minds and to fulfill their roles as listeners. All of us—and particularly our children—want to and need to be heard. A toddler begins to talk while his thinking is still in the realm of fantasy. He anxiously turns to his parents for expression and interpretation. A denial or ignoring of the child's world of fantasies in this period may be the most injurious to his future emotional development.

One way of stimulating healthy self-expression in a child is by being an attentive and sympathetic listener. It is essential that a child be encouraged to talk freely, to express his innermost ideas, feelings and wishes, and that we become receptive to his communications. For parents, listening in the early years of a child's growth depends not just on the fact of being quiet and attentive. Of even greater importance is the *conveyance* of a *sympathetic and wholehearted attitude of acceptance.*

Disturbed listening presupposes faulty personality development. Each newborn child has the capacity to listen effectively unless afflicted at birth with some organic hearing defect. This child, given a chance and a healthy parental soil, can develop normally and will fulfill his growth possibilities. His listening ability will grow in direct proportion to his state of emotional freedom and experiencing, to his degree of awareness as to what he is and where he is going, to the nature of his relationships to others and, finally, to his capacity to conceptualize realistically.

A child who lacks sympathetic listeners is driven to passive indulgence in movies, television, radio or reading comics. As he grows toward adolescence, he faces newer life stresses and problems that need attention, clarification and proper guidance. This crucial time, should a youngster find himself denied the sympathetic and understanding listening of his parents, might well be the origin of serious personality problems. With no one to help him by listening to his problems, he may be forced to seek less desirable outlets; what may result is what society has labeled "juvenile delinquency." A child who is the product of a home where listening and conversations are restricted or limited or one in which there are strained relationships between members of the family, is bound to suffer traumatic effects as a consequence.

The overprotective parent tends to keep the child from growing up or listening effectively and will choke whatever healthy independence there is to begin with in the child. He demands that obedience and discipline be one of forced submission and appeasement. The environmental tempo in this specific relationship is usually explosive and tempestuous. A child rarely knows what to expect when he confronts such a parent, what to say or when to listen. One moment he may be feverishly hugged, kissed, fondled or praised; again and under similar conditions, he will meet with harsh criticism or punishment.

Children cannot be muffled. Yet there are parents who insist upon this and so the child is subjected to one continual "shush." Children should be "seen but not heard." Communication is usually tense and filled with such strict or punitive responses as "do this," "don't do that," "you never listen," "shame on you," "you must," etc. One

103

can readily understand the frustration and forced rebellion that will develop in a child living in such a disturbing home.

A home which recognizes the mutual respect and responsibility of each and every member of its group does so by emphasizing both aspects of communication— namely, talking and listening. The environment in such a home is usually one in which its participants feel free to express all kinds of ideas, yet simultaneously develop an awareness for listening exchange and sympathetic understanding, both of which can only have a positive influence on the child's growth.

The perfectionistic parent, though similar in personality makeup to the overprotective parent, assumes somewhat different attitudes toward his children. Here we find a tendency to expect constant excellence, even perfection, in their children. Usually extremely ambitious for their children, such parents make excessive demands upon them, often pushing them far beyond their capacities in their lack of understanding or appreciation for the child's capacities, potentialities, talents or wants. The parental drive here is all toward abstract perfection, prestige and personal achievement.

In this particular parental milieu, a child's listening abilities may also be greatly disturbed. He soon feels that he must always be attentive and an exceptionally good listener. He must never allow himself to daydream or to forget what has been told to him. He must always comprehend his parents' words of wisdom. Never permitted to give signs of weakness, he is expected to stand up for his rights, fight his own battles, never complain and learn to become hard and calloused. In his performance he is expected to excel, and always to be on top.

The parents I have just briefly described are typical of those who do not listen effectively. We become accustomed to setting up patterns of thinking and hearing which act as screens of resistance between ourselves and our children. We are prejudiced, dogmatic, set in our ideas, and too often feel that our children should talk less and listen more. Our rationalization is that being older, we are also wiser.

Some parents become "half" listeners. They listen to their children with blank faces, giving the false impression of being attentive. This lack of personal involvement between parents and children often becomes the origin for feelings of inadequacy and rejection, and insofar as it disturbs holistic listening, it leads ultimately to a disruption in the parent-child relationship.

Furthermore parents who *force* their children to listen cause them to develop an inner automatic control system. In time these children when faced with painful emotional situations, learn to turn their listening mechanisms "on and off" instead of using them more spontaneously. They become either "forced listeners" who listen rebelliously or they develop into "partial-listeners," listening only when it suits their needs.

The period spent in school which every child in our particular culture undergoes can be of utmost significance in the development of the ability to listen. In our present educational setup we do our best to emphasize visual aids, yet discourage the use of ears. The blackboard, the use of mimeographed instructions and the constant verbal repetition of information and directions encourage the child not to listen attentively unless absolutely necessary.

In a study[4] at the University of Minnesota a few years ago, several hundred freshmen were tested for listening ability. The one hundred best and the one hundred poorest listeners were carefully studied through personal interviews, written questionnaires and several kinds of objective tests. Among other questions, the students were asked about their radio listening.

Some of the conclusions were: Of the poorest listeners, fewer than five per cent listened to programs requiring concentrated aural attention, programs comparable to *Meet the Press, America's Town Meeting of the Air, The Chicago Round Table* and *American Forum of the Air.* In fact, many of these students indicated that they were not even acquainted with the titles of these presentations.

The one hundred best listeners told of frequent listening to this type of radio program and expressed a liking for educational lectures in their home communities. The poor listeners hardly ever went to lectures, while the better listeners frequently attended.

In the adult, we discover further distortions and emotional disturbances in the areas of speaking and listening. An individual who feels basically divided experiences anxiety and an inner disorganization affecting his organism as a whole. Unable to preserve enough of his real self to express clearly or directly the true intent of his thoughts and feelings, he becomes increasingly confused and reacts poorly to his environment. He is not able to perform clearly or productively, with the result that objective reality situations become subjectively experienced with irrational emotions and in abnormal proportion to their true evaluative perspective. In the ultimate analysis, we find that instead of free-flowing spontaneous expression, a blocking, hesitant and confused form of communicative behavior ensues.

Because of their inner rigidities, fears and anxieties, these listeners dread the mutual exchange of ideas and beliefs. They listen only to what they feel they *should* be attentive to, blotting out larger areas of awareness and thus avoiding the basic truth involved in issues and situations. They are constantly suspicious and cautious about other people's reactions and set up emotional filters which disturb effective listening. Because of their hypersensitivity to criticism and rebuff, they are constantly on their guard and on the defensive. They listen with prejudiced opinions, preconceived notions, condemnations and cynical attitudes.

106

They fear facing or listening to the truth about themselves, and as a result their hearing becomes colored with absolute judgments, "black and white" evaluations and distorted emotional reactions.

Another point to be considered in listening is the fact that we cannot be aware of everything as it is or appears to be. We can only see and listen to the fullest extent of our individual capacities, remembering always that some degree of total awareness will be blotted out or missed in the final picture. From here on in, the process of listening and perceiving becomes a productive one only if we take whatever information we have heard and examine it for what it is without distortion, misinterpretation or conflicting affectation.

Confusion in relation to the process of listening comes about mainly when we place inhibitions and blockages in our path toward real understanding. Meaningful truth is not something we can gather from the outside. It comes primarily from an inner state of direct perception, real awareness, understanding and the capacity to feel and readily accept things as *they are*. To know exactly what *is*—the real, the actual—without interpreting it, without condemning or justifying it, is surely the beginning of wisdom.

Freud assigned a special place to the auditory lobe and to listening in his early structural formulation of the neurosis. As a result, we now assume a definite and subconscious connection *between the word and the command*. Thus for a child, an adult's prohibition may become his "voice of conscience" which in turn will directly reflect his future inner inhibitions and self-imposed psychic restrictions. Enlarging on this further, Isakower refers to the auditory sphere as the "nucleus of the superego," his premise being that we learn from speech which reaches us through the entire "auditory sphere," i.e., the acoustic apparatus from end organ to psychic representation.

107

Through this we take in the word sounds, ultimately formulating the attitudes of our environment, so creating an inner observing and criticizing institution. Thus the auditory mechanism keeps us oriented in our world of conduct just as the adjacent and embryologically similar apparatus does in the world of space.

Disturbances in listening are usually expressed in what we commonly refer to as *distractions*. When we are troubled, conflicted or tense, we place blockages and screens in the path of our true perception and we talk compulsively so as not to listen. This evasion becomes a substitute for feeling and emotion. The result is that we listen as we experience ourselves at the time—disorganized, confused, disinterested—and with half an ear.

The following are some of the blockages which interfere with effective or productive listening:—

1) *Disturbances in productivity:*—The use of words or phrases which are clumsy, circumstantial or strongly intellectual in variety tends to interfere with the free flow of conversation. People who speak in terms of absolutes and rigid "black-or-white" terms tend to provoke inappropriate feedback responses and confused or blank expressions from their listeners. The listener unable to comprehend clearly the meaning of the original message responds with difficulty. His reply usually does not fit the circumstances, nor is it relevant and thus does not match the initial statement. Or, the reply may be exaggerated because it is an expression of anger or colored with politeness in a timid individual. The total response of the listener under these conditions is usually characterized by a lack of flexibility, a forced control, remoteness, extreme redundancy and loss of information.

2) *Subject Responses of Frustration:*—According to Ruesch, for most people's experience, "a balance has to be found between adequacy of reply and introduction of new topics, between self-expression and adaptation to the situation,

108

between repetition and new formulation, and between flexibility and rigidity."[5] This balance which is geared to the human being's tolerance for social stimulation and his need for expression and action is frequently upset. The result is frustration which can become the foremost criterion of disturbed communication.

People *need to communicate* in order to relate to those about them. When this communication is interfered with, group participation becomes defective and conversation is disturbed. Interpersonal relationships break down. Frustrated we become tense, restless, irritable, hostile and resentful. Communication as a whole has broken down. We cannot reason with one another, levels of agreement cannot be reached and further signs of frustration appear. We begin to feel excluded from the group and our listening capacities start to decrease. We become poor listeners, listening in a machine-like automatic sense, with our ears instead of our hearts.

In *How to Talk with People*, Irving Lee reports the observations he made as an objective observer at two hundred meetings of boards and committees. He found that the major types of trouble people have in trying to talk with each other, all reflect in one way or another some sort of "jamming" of the feedback. People seem to be far more driven to talk to each other than to listen to each other, and when they do listen, the kind of response they give the speaker and the reaction of the speaker to this feedback, are often colored with emotions of resentment, self-defensiveness, suspicion and confusion. Group communication is disrupted by the lack of cooperation, mutuality or sincerity.

When we are conflicted, as has been said, we block and inhibit many of the true messages and communications which seek to emerge from within ourselves. We become anxious and find it difficult to listen to and to feel our real innermost thoughts, beliefs or wishes. Our listening is numbed as we find the distortions of our state of being expressed in bodily symptoms of general tiredness or restlessness. In other words, conflicting ideas and feelings of a strong and painful nature which should be felt consciously are silenced instead of mental mechanisms. They are forced to find their expressions through a kind of "organ" language.

Physical complaints of neurotic origin are only bodily expressions of psychological conflict. When communication is disturbed, any vital threat to the safety of either the speaker or listener may set in motion a powerful response in the autonomic nervous system, disturbances known as psychosomatic ailments of the heart, endocrine glands, skeletal musculature, digestive system, even—in instances—of such severe shock as death. Although what actually passes between speaker and listener is nothing more than air and light waves which in themselves as manifestations of physical force are weak and perfectly harmless, the reception of verbal messages at times may result in serious consequences to the listener.

The language of this body or "organ" language is astonishingly well described in everyday popular phrases. For example, when we hear something unpleasant or something that we don't want to hear, we speak of not being able to "swallow" it. When we want to "shut off" or "turn off" an unpleasant verbal message, we frequently feel a constriction in the chest or belly, indicating that we have something we would like to get rid of by talking it out. When we listen to something "we can't stomach," we feel nausea, revealing an inclination to vomit away our difficulties. We "burn up" or "blow our tops" when we hear something that annoys us; as we listen compulsively, we open our ears wide, accepting everything— truths, half-truths or fiction. In so doing, we use up so much energy that we have little left for constructive use and thus we constantly find ourselves tired and restless.

These and many other similar examples are indications that the body has a peculiar language of its own through which it conveys feelings and meanings it is unable to listen to or verbalize and thus healthily abstract to higher and more productive bodily levels.

In hysteria we find a dramatic form of expression of organ language. In hysterical deafness, for instance, the individual is faced with an unbearable or unacceptable reality, which he unconsciously avoids experiencing by resorting to symptom formation. When strong emotions interfere with what we want to hear, our peace is disturbed and listening becomes impossible or, in the case of deafness, blotted out altogether.

In hysterical deafness, we hear something that opposes what we feel we *should* hear in the form of our most deeply rooted prejudices, notions, convictions and values. We thus become afraid and anxiously set up a block in the path of our listening. We develop mental barriers which interfere with our ability to be open-minded and to listen with humility and understanding. Finally, hysterical deafness represents an attempt to satisfy two conflicting drives—the wish to assert one's self and express hostility openly and the opposing need to be accepted, loved and thought of as being "nice" by the group. The result of these contradictory emotional pulls is one of marked emotional and physical stress, inhibition, paralysis and blocking of a person's whole being—including his listening.

For *real communication*, there are *no barriers between listening and speaking*. As Oliver, the noted speech expert, recently wrote, "For the real master of communication . . . listening and talking are interwoven . . . like the warp and the woof of a piece of cloth. When he is listening, he is standing at the threshold of his companion's mind; and when he is talking, he invites his auditor to stand at the doorway of his own thought."[7]

In contradistinction, the poor listener is likely to be a

111

poor talker as well. When others are talking, his mind wanders, he becomes distracted and takes in only half of what others have to say. Because of his prejudices, fixed notions and dogmatic beliefs, his responses assume a coloring of vagueness, remoteness and superficiality. He aims his remarks over and around his audience, rather than straight to the heart of the matter. To sum it up, the effective listener is one who *uses* silence as he uses talk—with an eager, alive and generous desire to share.

References

1, 2. Ralph G. Nichols and Leonard A. Stevens: *Are You Listening?* New York, McGraw-Hill, 1957, p. 4.

3. *Ibid.*, p. 6.

4. *Ibid.*, p. 205.

5. Jurgen Ruesch: *Disturbed Communication.* New York, Norton & Company, 1957, p. 44.

6. Irving Lee: *How to Talk with People.* New York, Harper & Brothers, 1951.

7. Robert T. Oliver: "One Man's Opinion." *Today's Speech,* Vol. V, No. 4, Nov. 1957.

Listening with a Modest Ear

Speech finely framed delighteth the ears.

Those who listen with a "modest" ear usually do so in a passive and sentimental way. They are what I refer to as the "compulsive nodders," i.e., those who will nod and shake their heads in agreement so as to give the impression of being always attentive and understanding. They may be likened to Caesar's barber, whom Plutarch called a "really busy listening fellow!"

To a large extent, we live today in an age of conformity. From early childhood we are trained to sit back passively and allow facts from the outside world to pour into our ears with little effort or involvement on our part. We are content mostly to be habitual listeners and permit ourselves to be influenced by some of the great inventions of our time—radio, movies, television.

If a speaker be an authority or a person of prominence in the public eye, we automatically assume that we can listen to and safely follow his judgments and pronouncements without bothering to use our own critical faculties. We evaluate the intent and importance of what we hear not so much as to its basic content but in relation to the degree to which we are impressed and affected. Too frequently this appeal depends on the speaker's external appearance, his poise, his delivery and his ability to avoid issues which will disturb or antagonize his listeners more than on what he is actually saying.

113

Too many of us blindly accept the so-called influential speakers of our day—the politicians, college professors, preachers, newspapermen and television commentators. We listen to these speakers with total acceptance and respect and rarely do we question their ability to communicate effectively. It is their intent—one might say their business—to persuade and hypnotize those of us who are more than ready to participate passively by having ideas handed down to us. And they are successful to the extent that we swear by them, cheer for them, get into arguments defending what they have said. We are often content to accept facts at face value simply because they have been endorsed by someone of importance. Yet how often do we ask ourselves what is actually being said and if it has any real meaning for us? How often do we stop to consider how we actually *feel* about what we have just heard? We prefer to be habitual listeners who listen automatically to sounds and noises with which we have little active self-involvement or real perception.

No doubt all of you have come into contact at some time or other with these "compulsive nodders" in your own conversational groups. Since they seek an audience to satisfy their own neurotic needs, their main emphasis is in the direction of their wish to please, to receive approbation and applause. This wish to placate others, to find good in everything, to be always accepted, usually disturbs the pattern of conversation and causes it to acquire a coquettish and seductive tone. Conversation groups built around this pollyanna principle are little more than mutual admiration societies.

Listeners of this sort take a peculiar delight in feeling that people can pour their hearts out to them. They take pride in believing that, unlike other selfish and inattentive listeners, they have the capacity "to take an earful." In the process of their listening, they become extremely apologetic, self-effacing and humble. Like the timid soul, they bend stiffly forward almost as though they were about to dart at their speaker. Little does the speaker know that his impact on such a listener is lost in this shrinking process. For in their compulsive need to appear *always* nice, overattentive and sympathetic, these listeners perforce lose contact with the actual verbal situation. So much concern is given to *how* they are listening and reacting to the speaker that they miss out on what is actually being said. In their urgency to arouse a favorable response from their speakers, they are too often much more finicky about how they appear to others than about the clarity, validity or basic content of the message.

Compliant listeners may be compared to what Clifton Fadiman[1] refers to as the "enfeebling intensifiers." In conversational groups they are the ones who make constant use of the handy "okay" or its variants, or the richly varied *y-p* series: *yap*, *yahp*, *yep*, *yip*, *yop* and *yup*. At other times in order to dramatize more firmly their nod of approval, they use such cliches as "definitely," "you can say that again," "I know just what you mean" and the truer nicety, "you're so right."

There are others in this category who will take great pride in being able to say that above all they like to "get the facts." This often becomes a facade to cover their inner fear of arriving at true understanding or intimacy by appearing to be overly attentive and alert. The truth of the matter is that in the attempt to give the appearance of being a good listener and in trying to memorize every single fact that is spoken, the true intent of the message becomes lost. Memorizing what is said is not an effective way to listen.

Though listeners of this variety give the impression of listening with intense interest and curiosity, they become easily distracted when the discussion becomes too involved or demands the use of extra listening efforts. External distractions such as noise, other people talking, changing temperatures in the room, or some indication of disinterest shown by the other person, immediately set up a difficult listening situation and make it "too hard" for them to hear. They like to speak in a whisper, mouth their sounds and at times are difficult to comprehend, yet from those listening they demand absolute attention, no distractions and complete understanding.

For communication to be effective, its network has to be functionally organized and the flow of messages has to be adapted to its capacity. If one portion is overloaded and another is not used, breakdown of the communication system is a possibility.

In the dependent listener, the need to hear and digest everything that is being said can easily lead to an overloading and jamming of the communication network. In their attempts to achieve the impossible in listening capacity, these listeners create more messages than can be effectively heard and thus become too difficult to handle or comprehend satisfactorily. The tolerance limits for listening become overextended, most stimuli become too intense and buffer systems fail to function properly. The result is a disorganized communication system. For example, children who are exposed to a continuous barrage of demands and expectations from their parents tend to develop similar disturbances in listening. Parents of this sort are unaware of the child's limited capacity to absorb such stimulation. What then occurs is that, in their attempts to satisfy their parents, these children may be driven to becoming "compulsive nodders" or they will learn to respond with superficial gestures or words.

Furthermore, these listeners, because of their over-dependency needs, live vicariously through the opinions, wishes and feelings of others. Their main concern depends not so much on the exchange of information and cooperative interaction as on the protective actions of others. They have, as Ruesch puts it, "the naive and

116

magic belief that the other person's physical and mental state is identical with their own. Therefore, they treat messages as if they were transmitted within one and the same matrix or neural network, and they do not know that interpersonal messages have to be repeatedly recodified and translated."[2] They cannot, as a result, utilize the perceived effect of their actions upon others and are therefore unable to correct the image they possess of themselves. Their need for lasting acceptance and unconditional approval compels them to treat everyone with whom they come into contact as insiders. In listening, they immediately place all messages on a primitive or infantile level and so are unable to deal with abstract matters.

In communicative exchange these people find it difficult to acknowledge another person's statements directly. They rarely decipher the messages of others correctly, nor are they able to make their own intent known in return. Their ears become attuned not so much to situational facts or statements as to their need to protect themselves from feeling tension and to fulfill their dependency needs. Their fear of intruding upon others or disturbing interpersonal contact causes them to engulf most sounds just so that they may be thought of as pleasant and charming. In so doing, they make an implied claim upon others for protective action and surrendering love.

Behavioristically the "modest listener" is predominantly a self-effacing person. In his relations with others, he exhibits in most of his responses, including those of speaking and listening, compulsive expressions of compliancy, timidity and dependency. Given to going out of his way to make himself appear smaller than others, to be dependent upon them and to appear modest and unobtrusive, he is the exact opposite of the expansive person who glorifies himself and cultivates in himself anything that gives him a sense of omnipotence.

The self-effacing person lives with a diffuse sense of failure because of his inability to be accepted and liked as he feels he *should* be. Inwardly he constantly considers and judges himself inferior, worthless and beneath notice and will seek to constrict himself in most areas of his life. For fear of intruding upon others or appearing too arrogant or presumptuous, he will suppress in himself any reaction that might seem to signify ambition, vindictiveness, assertiveness, or a seeking after his own advantage.

Such people also feel and experience their environment as potentially dangerous and of an impending attacking nature. In place of any genuine or resourceful attempt to meet disturbing situations, they respond to fear by becoming basically anxious, helpless and apprehensive. They rarely counterattack directly, but instead will shrink in attitude, plead helplessness and place themselves at the mercy of others by seeking dependency or achieving protection through a form of surrendering love.

Such a person communicates on what I call a "dependent or comprising level," accepting at face value what is said to him, rarely questioning who is speaking to him or what is being said. He listens in an automatic sense, as though messages were being relayed to him through a public amplifier. It is not important to him at the time that he question the validity of what is said to him just as long as the speaker is being listened to with absorption by his audience as he speaks with impressive authority. For this reason, the basic meaning of the message or the listener's relation to the communicative setup takes a secondary position in the actual situation.

Consider, for instance, how often and how many of us listen to a sermon, a lecture, a piece of music or political talk without concerning ourselves overly much with the moral messages involved or attempting to take part in what we are hearing with an active ear. In place of involving ourselves wholly and listening with as much

118

thought as possible at the moment, we sit back passively, giving the impression of being good listeners. And ironically, at the same time we feel compelled to give the impression that we have fully understood what was conveyed to us, that we are satisfied and that effective communication has taken place. However, we fool only ourselves. Our awkward and forced actions and our parrot-like responses will give us away and the *feeling* tone becomes one of tension, confusion and estrangement. The communication system has broken down and both parties leave it with too little basic understanding or satisfaction having been derived.

The self-effacing person *communicates by complacency* instead of *by conviction or assertion*. His fear of meeting with the disapproval of others compels him to listen with an expression of agreement. In meeting someone new, he rarely initiates the discussion, hoping the other person will take over, make the first crucial move and assume the main responsibility. This will also give him ample time and opportunity to set in motion his own apparatus of compliancy. He can now put on his loving puppy expression, open his eyes wide, assume an expression of being content and affable, and so set about winning over those about him with his seducing charm. His ears automatically opened wide, all sounds and noises are permitted to enter and yet little true perception or discrimination takes place. The prime motive of such a listener is to be seductive, modest and lovable. What he is listening to or whether he understands or is being understood is not essential.

Once the machinery of compliancy is set in motion, the listener with a modest ear is no longer functioning effectively. His audience appears vague, distant and hazy, he himself feels alienated, and the whole communicative effect begins to disintegrate and disorganize. Levels of tension increase and accelerate and as the speaker is forced to make more vigorous attempts to activate and restore balance in the communicative situation, the listener in his own chaotic way tries more earnestly to draw in all that is being said, yet not lose the personal approval of his speaker. Depending on the compulsive and indiscriminate needs of both speaker and listener, the intensity and disorganization of such situations will last from a few seconds to a number of exhausting hours and will vary from feelings of slight discomfort to heightened anxiety or even panic.

The self-effacing listener is not one to want or seek differences, controversies or arguments. His need for peaceful coexistence and harmonious agreement is a compulsive aspect of his make-up. In listening to others, he avoids messages or communicative responses which will give rise to personal discord or disfavor. Should he wish to introduce his own comments into the discussion, he usually blots out such thoughts and becomes instead the understanding and agreeable one. His ears are quick to catch the so-called pleasantries and social niceties; and in turn his own language to a large extent becomes one of accord. As he listens, his main emphasis is on nodding compulsively in agreement; and wherever he can, he injects such cliches as "I agree with you entirely," "there is no doubt that you are perfectly right," "that is what I thought, too," or "if you say so, it is all right with me."

Disturbed listeners give to the "noises" they hear special meanings that will fit their own neurotic solutions. The unduly timid, compliant, self-effacing person, hypersensitive to the world he lives in, feels easily rejected, rebuffed and hurt by being made the target of harsh, unfair or insulting remarks. However, because of his tendency to distort words and misinterpret many verbal situations, he makes himself still more vulnerable. Since he feels he lives in a pollyanna-like world, he often attributes destructive, critical or even sarcastic evaluations to harmless messages which he feels are aimed directly at him. He equates words with things, giving them special meanings. Because he feels so invaded, he is frequently prone to disregard the actuality that another person communicates to him, to distort the specific word-contexts, and to interpret them as what he feels the speaker meant to say. For this reason, his hearing becomes disturbed and colored with feelings of hostility, abused reactions and accusations.

Again, he rarely attempts to modify his wave lengths or to remove the static he hears. Instead his taboo on aggression or assertion makes him all the more timid and unobtrusive. At this point, to offset an attack he may try to placate his opponent by an overeager admission of "not having heard too well." He may now say: "You are quite right, I must have misunderstood you;" "I should have heard you the first time;" "I should be a more sympathetic listener." Or if he is hurt or angry enough, he may revert to the opposite strategy of attempting to create embarrassment and a defensive reaction in his persecutor by saying: "Your words have stunned my ears;" "I just don't have the strength to listen any more;" "What you have said is most unfair; no one has ever said such things to me before."

The predominantly self-effacing person is in constant dread of appearing superior to others in any situation. In communication, he usually feels himself smaller, inferior, insignificant and unimportant in relation to his speaker. When listening, he feels compelled to absorb every minute sound that comes from his audience, for fear of appearing too dull, inattentive or just bored. He usually remains in the background, speaks only when asked to or when directly questioned.

Should he have a point to make or an idea to contribute to an issue about which he feels strongly, he may deny its expression in the open. He may even make himself believe that he heard incorrectly to begin with and therefore think his opinion would have little effect. Or he may rationalize his action to remain silent because he has decided that what he was about to say was not really important at all. What he is really avoiding in his impeded listening and in his fear of speaking is the possibility of causing friction or provoking hostility in others.

Still further, such a listener may assume a stoic front and attempt to make others feel ashamed for his silence. In this situation he tells himself that since most other people are cold and harsh and therefore do not have the same understanding and patience he feels he has when listening, he would prefer to remain uncommunicative. In so doing, he can make future claims on his audience for their fullest attention, utter patience with him and no criticism of his remarks. In the final analysis what he would like to achieve is his own image of himself as both a charming and modest listener and a seducing orator.

Our compliant person is constantly on the alert for soft and endearing terms. In communicative exchange his need to be liked and to be thought of as charming causes him to ignore most messages and instead listen for sounds which appear to be soft and melodious. He enjoys being hypnotized by the whispers and sweet nothings of conversation, avoiding any free exchange of opinion. To be involved in the latter may mean friction or the criticism he hopes to avoid at all costs.

The timid listener, because of his shrinking qualities, leans over backward to shun anything he considers forward, conceited or aggressive. Afraid to chance his own opinions or convictions, he gives in easily to everyone else's ideas. Should the need arise, he will find it almost impossible to defend himself when he has been criticized unjustly.

There is much hostility in such a listener, but he is rarely able to show it. Inwardly he prefers to see himself as a person whose wings have been clipped, one too

122

crippled to be a good fighter. Moreover, due to his terror lest anyone be hostile, he is compelled to be loved and to avoid friction with others at all cost. He would rather give in and suffer under the pretense of being understanding and forgiving. In so doing he is able to glorify in himself the lovable qualities of goodness, generosity, humility and nobility.

The smaller such a person makes himself appear, the more will his audience prey upon him. Aggressive speakers take delight in cornering such a listener for their own destructive needs. They talk down to him, shout at him and intimidate him with their words. They thrill in watching him tremble and shake his head in agreement as he appears to give a speaker his full attention. Such a listener suits an aggressive person's needs because he does not dare interrupt or disturb the communicative exchange and so the speaker is able to control the situation without fear that he will be questioned, criticized or disturbed.

The self-effacing person is spellbound by speakers he considers as strong, assertive and influential. He becomes infatuated with these qualities both aggressive and expansive which he feels are missing in himself. A captive audience, his need to charm and seduce others compels him to listen. He feels no free choice in his relation to others and thus feels inescapably imprisoned. Though others may impose the need to listen, he does not object but will become instead a "forced" listener. He will always try to appear polite, look at the speakers with dreamy eyes and give the impression of being completely attentive and alert, whereas in reality he is distant, anxious, and confused, his hearing is disturbed and colored with static.

This same individual is torn between the need on the one hand to be outstanding and aggressive, and on the other by the need to be approved, admired and blindly loved. In such a dilemma, he is prone to feel conflicted in thought, feeling and action. His hearing and speech both become colored with inhibitions and hesitations, indicative of all the conflicts and their accompanying attempts to restore order to his disorganized personality.

Listening is most effective when one is closest to being his real self. The effective listener is one who feels himself equal in any communicative exchange. He must know himself able to express his opinions openly and to meet justifiable criticism, anger or hostility. On the other hand, a person who feels divided and disorganized is unable to make use of all his resources. His entire organism, especially his hearing, becomes defective in function. The communication system breaks down as messages are poorly received and erroneously transmitted to others. As a result, both speaker and listener become tense and anxious, feedback systems become jammed, misunderstanding occurs, and the ultimate situation is one of confusion and misunderstanding, anger and hostility. Furthermore there are those who want to feel hostility toward others and to arouse discord, and at the same time to appear calm, gentle, unperturbed, and to express themselves with words that are soft, kind and endearing. These listeners who wish to live in a state of perpetual euphoria are prone to fail realistically and to suffer from the effects of this failure.

The self-effacing individual as a result of his conflicting and contradictory attitudes suffers many adverse consequences. He is basically at odds with himself and others. In the specific communicative situation, his disturbances become reflected both in his verbalizations and in his inability to listen effectively. His fear of facing facts or situations in their true perspective makes him listen poorly and distort true evaluations. Finally, as a means of avoiding anxiety and further inner chaos, he will feel compelled to manipulate the true meaning of his messages, transforming them with all sorts of magical colorings to make them conform to his specific neurotic needs. Ultimately barriers are set up in the path of arriving at any real understanding of the meaningful act.

To listen effectively, it is imperative that we be free and spontaneous enough to be selective in the communicative situation and not feel coerced into interpreting what we feel was meant to be said. The tendency to disregard actual word-contexts and give false subjective meanings to messages, disturbs and alters the whole communication network, giving rise to personality disintegration and feelings of tension, apprehension, confusion, anger or hostility. True communication can only arise as we are increasingly able to set aside our inner fears, prejudices, condemnations and resentments, thus permitting a freer exchange of thought, wishes and opinions. Messages will then be understood in their real context—as they are *meant to be*, not as we feel *they should be*. As more levels of agreement are finally reached, feelings of tension and anxiety lessen, and both intrapsychic and interpersonal relations improve and a healthy communicative exchange will take place.

References

1. Clifton Fadiman: *Party of One*. New, York, The World Publishing Company, 1955, p. 440.
2. Jurgen Ruesch: *Disturbed Communication*. New York, W. W. Norton & Company, 1957, p. 118.

Listening with a Rebellious Ear

Empty barrels make the most noise

ANOTHER type of listener is one who listens with what we shall call "rebellious" ears. In this category we have the chatterboxes who make a fetish of talking incessantly, who seldom listen when you speak to them. Their compulsive need to be the center of attraction and to be the sole speakers in a group, makes them restless and disinterested when others talk. We often find them at cocktail parties or social gatherings where such people rarely listen to what is said to them, let their attention wander constantly, and with clucking tongues give out with that meaningless variety of talk known as blah. The late humorist Robert Benchley once dramatized this situation most effectively by circulating about at a large talky party, making idiotic statements such as "Tonight it may snow if the whistle stops." Few of those present were aware that he was deliberately uttering nonsense.

The rebellious individual listens in a defensive and annoying manner. He is rarely enthusiastic about what a person has to say to him, is impatient, and interferes at regular intervals. He must be the master of the conversation and have *the last word*. His own egocentricity compels him to quote himself continually and to make numerous references about himself, his world, his ideas and beliefs—all to the exclusion of anyone else's.

In the role of the interrogator, he will become defiant and ask questions with the "hot-seat" technique used by TV interviewer Mike Wallace. He rarely puts others at ease in conversation, has an unfriendly attitude, is defensive and, by showing a lack of genuine interest, does nothing to establish any feeling of rapport. In his urgency to take over the discussion, he has no time to listen attentively to what is being said. He has what may be compared to a "one way tuner equipment, with an all transmitter and no receptor mechanism." Eager to defend himself and to have that last word, he listens only to the first dozen or so words, and from then on he is involved in his forward attack.

In his listening, this kind of person is rarely interested in what others have to say. He puts on an act in seeming to be attentive, yet he seldom listens to a person as a whole being. He is interested chiefly in the surface facts, and in readying himself for bringing forth his own arguments in defense. When something difficult or penetrating is discussed, he passes it up, ignores its value content, or dismisses it as being too complex or unnecessary. Or feeling pinned down or pressed into listening, he is likely to become resentful and detach himself completely from the conversation, by prematurely dismissing what the speaker has to say as uninteresting. In so doing, he is able to avoid any exposure of himself by appearing aloof, indifferent and disinterested.

The rebellious listener lives by the use of "hit-'em-hard" tactics with which he reinforces his way of life by adhering to the philosophy of the jungle—"an eye for an eye and a tooth for a tooth." His one main orientation in life is the attainment of prestige and success, and therefore he shies away from any resemblance to softer feelings for either himself or others. In listening to others, he has little time for the details or frailties of everyday living. It is his conviction that most of his friends and associates are too soft these days, and have nothing to do but chatter and talk about foolish nothings. He has no time for chit-chat and will demand that his speaker come down to basic issues and get to the real facts. Social niceties or preliminary conversational warm-ups are just a waste of time to him and a way of avoiding the truth. His one major concern in talking or listening to others is what is he getting out of a situation, and "to hell with the next person." He takes pride in believing that in this hard and practical world, everyone must take care of himself or succumb.

People who consider themselves as being always right of necessity become poor listeners. Because of their blindness in seeing a situation as a means to an end rather than on the basis of its intrinsic worth, they listen only to "half-truths." Their ears are closed to the gentler feelings or emotional intonations of life. The need to place a premium on such qualities as hardness, shrewdness, cynicism and toughness makes the aggressive person feel justified in acting rebelliously and disparagingly toward others. The sound of soft and tender words or the warmth of sentimentality frightens them, for their greatest fear is that in being thought soft they will be compelled to lose their armor of hardness and so will fall prey to others.

As he listens to others, the aggressive individual will demand absolute admiration, full acceptance and blind obedience from his companions. In turn, when he speaks he feels that he should be and *is* the authority. He will stubbornly refuse to listen to anything that may question his position of omnipotence. When cornered with the truth, he becomes stubborn, hostile and highly reluctant to face the issues at hand squarely and honestly. He will use all sorts of maneuvers to distract and foil his audience with vacuities, one-sided misrepresentations, and then when he feels the moment to be ripe, he will explode his bomb, thereby attempting to catch his listener by surprise. Moreover he takes pleasure in belittling his opponent and will scorn him openly.

A prejudiced speaker, and known to be a poor listener, he yet does not want to give anybody else a chance to talk. Because of his fear of finding himself in any position but that of superiority, he is driven to becloud most issues and distort their true meanings to suit his own needs. Should he be shown to be in error, he will become arrogantly disdainful. If questioned, he will consciously avoid having to listen nor will he try to share ideas. Instead he becomes immediately defensive, seeking to outsmart, outwit, or outtalk anyone who may differ with him. He sees everything in rigid, absolute, two-valued orientations. Everything is either good or bad, right or wrong. And, of course, he is *always* right. Should his listeners appear not to be responsive enough, he will then resort to the use of words and phrases that can only arouse strong and antagonistic feelings. He thus is able either to make himself the master of a situation, or he will stubbornly limit himself to a rebellious form of anticipation.

This same individual takes a great pride in believing he has sharp ears. In his illusion that he never misses a trick, he strengthens his neurotic position of omnipotence by appearing to be keen, alert, different, unique and opposite from others. As he continues to listen, he distorts many of the facts in order that he may make them fit his own frame of reference. At such times where he may feel he is bored or is no longer the center of attraction, he will try to distract his speaker with an array of confusing and ambiguous questions. Once his speaker is sufficiently weakened, he then moves in in an effort to regain prominence in the discussion by turning on his entire arsenal of intellectual weapons—memorized quotations, hidden facts, or data of any sort usually missed by the average eye and ear. To his way of thinking, any form of strategy which gives him the upper hand in a communicative situation is a legitimate counter against his greatest fear—exposure as being in the wrong or intellectually inferior to others.

The rebellious listener is for the most part a *person of action*. His fear of being alone and his inability to evaluate his own self-worth, compels him to be constantly with others. In communicative exchange, there is almost never a homogeneous network, for he prevents himself from observing and sharing mutually with others, by talking all the time. He rarely respects the opinions of others, is a fragmentary listener, and functions only when he is the center of attention. Most of his energies are divided when conversing with others, and as a result he creates many distractions in the path of his listening. His need to grasp the advantage over others and his fear of being intellectually inferior to them makes him use most of his listening capacity to gain a momentary superiority and an opportunity to control the situation. The result is that such a person listens only to that which he feels will strengthen his neurotic hold and thus the exchange will promote little real growth or positive feedback relay. In his struggle to impress others and be thought of as omnipotent, his performance as a listener becomes less skillful but more impressive to the audience.

In his drive to achieve this mastery and control, the rebellious person of necessity pushes others away from himself and so will feel excluded from life in general. He is blind to the simple truth that it is his own suspiciousness, hostility and arrogance toward others that has created this state of forced exclusion. Because of his mistrust of his own words, he does not trust the words of other people, and believes that everyone is out to show him up. He thinks he has the right to tell others exactly what he thinks, yet becomes indignant should others seek to advise or caution him. Although he is too *proud* to listen to others, he will become hostile and infuriated with those he feels have no personal interest in his own welfare. He cannot imagine that anyone might relate to him without an ulterior motive in mind. His omnipotent picture of himself as vain and powerful remains unaffected by verbal intercourse.

In groups, this type of listener utilizes most of his energies and tactics toward assuming leadership over his audience. He will resort to being witty, the jokester of the crowd, and to any other communicative strategy which will give him the upper hand. His narcissistic make-up compels him to talk inconsistently and incessantly, with little connection at times to the subject at hand or with little consideration for others or perception problem as a whole. He is in fact so driven in this direction that he often fails to see that this logorrhea of his irritates and disturbs his listeners. His fear of being left open and exposed to attack from others may be so intense at times that he becomes insensitive and blind to his own shortcomings.

A person of this sort, because of his egocentric needs is engrossed in his own needs and feelings to the exclusion of those of others. He believes himself so unique, wonderful and far superior to others that listening to others is considered as a humble and considerate act. He deludes himself with the idea that he really loves people, that he is kind, understanding and generous, and so he will snatch at every opportunity to flatter and praise others. The truth of the matter is that he actually has contempt for others, and he will rarely permit himself to keep his ears open to their wishes, feelings or desires. He listens only to so much, and only to such facts as he can assimilate without encountering anxiety or danger to his god-like image of himself. He will appear to be attentive and give the semblance of being a good listener, providing he in return is given superiority and unconditional acceptance in the communicative exchange, no matter how much he may actually interfere with others' rights or wishes.

Because of his urgency to interfere and take command in conversation, this individual is of necessity a poor listener. He rarely listens since his thoughts are always one step further than those of his speaker. He acts prematurely, does not listen to all of the facts presented, and proceeds to evaluate by making snap judgments in terms of absolute and rigid values. He tends to generalize from insufficient information, antagonizes his speaker by constant interruptions and disagreements, and for the most part keeps his audience on the defensive. When a situation calls for evaluation, he cannot remain silent or reflect for the moment on a given problem. Instead he is compelled to talk and to transmit *his* ideas or feelings on the matter, just so that he can draw the attention away from someone else and regain control in the group. The end result however is that he will talk or act before he has made a sound decision, repeating traditional patterns of verbal action which will distort the true evaluation of the situation.

Due to this basic instability, this attitude of always being suspicious and doubtful of others in verbal exchange, his ears as he listens to others become attuned to any revealing facts which may substantiate victimized feelings of his. He is alert to anything said or implied which may give him an opening for venting his vindictiveness, his arrogance, his belief that those about him are at heart selfish, crooked and dishonest. He uses his listening capacities not to get at the true meaning of facts or situations, but to justify his own aggressive tactics and need for mastery. He will rudely interrupt or disagree with others when they are talking, but within himself any questioning, assertion or disagreements of his opinions, become threats to his pride, and thus a matter of destruction. What he fails to see or accept in the listening exchange is that others are also human beings who also have sensitive feelings. In his role as *master*, he feels only that all others are inferior to himself, and for this reason he is concerned only in the direction of his own welfare.

The rebellious listener in his attempts to assume control of the speaking situation, ignores and denies the feelings and rights of others. In listening, he rarely gives his full interest or attention and in his replies uses words to destroy any initiative that does not come from his side. He will use any trick to distract and throw off guard those who now have become his listeners. During the moments when he has to listen—and this he does not enjoy—he busies himself constantly with his tie, eyeglasses, rubbing his chin. Should his speaker insist upon cornering him, he will put forth a verbal attack, cynically criticize his imagined foe, or sit back with sophisticated disdain. In each verbal maneuver, he imagines himself to be the master of the situation, painfully subjecting himself to the frailties of his audience. He can only be enlightened and stimulated to life when he is successful in twisting the discussion to his way of thinking and when he can emerge as the brilliant and seducing orator. Woe betide any member of his audience who appears bored, disinterested or who denies him full and absolute attention. From his god-like pulpit, his listeners should be reverent and humble in receiving his words of wisdom.

Listening to be effective must be directed and selective. We as listening humans are conditioned to select and accept only those things which are pleasurable to our ears and do not disturb our emotions. If something is said which comes too close to our own personal emotional difficulties, we then become anxious, blocked, fearful and prone to experience difficulties in our auditive reception. Distractions in the path of our listening occur for the most part when we do not understand, when we feel frightened emotionally, or when we are at odds with our speakers.

The neurotic individual because of his egocentric make-up is in constant need of praise and recognition. When listening his ears are ever on the alert for words of admiration and glorification. He believes such recognition is his due and he will grow indignant if it is not forthcoming. Concomitantly when listening to others, his capacity to be sensitive to others or to give credit when it is earned, is extremely limited.

For such a person as hostile and isolated as he makes himself, it is essential that he not need or depend upon others. He thus develops a definite pride in his own god-like self-sufficiency. In conversational groups, he will change—depending on his moods—from a position equivalent to that of toastmaster to that of an aloof, disinterested onlooker. Should he be listening to someone else and not understand or follow the presenting trend of thought, he is often too proud to ask for clarification. On the other hand he will make every attempt to appear intelligent and will depend upon his luck and his vigilant strategy to outwit his speaker and to pull himself through the dilemma. This he desperately needs to achieve, for he relies upon only his intellect for the mastery of life. Hence, for such a person it is essential that he be always right when in communication with others, that he appear alert, that he have both foresight and an appearance of invincible strength.

Living with unresolved conflicts involves a devastating waste of energies expended not only on the conflicts themselves but also on all the roundabout attempts to remove these conflicts. It is no wonder then that the aggressive individual can never utilize all of his energies constructively nor direct them toward any one wholehearted purpose. Instead he becomes a human being divided, a division which encompasses all his senses including that of listening. His belief that he is god-like and his craving for perfection in any endeavor leads to a scattering of energies and interest. In his continued need to fortify his neurotic superstructure, he will find himself entangled in a web of conflicting feelings and thoughts which will create much inner confusion, distortion of interest and impaired concentration. All of these disturbances can only lead ultimately to distractions and poor listening.

A person who lacks real inner balance or a sense of being, will of necessity feel tense, strained, defensive, hostile and pressured. In communicative exchange, he will appear under control, on guard, suspicious and alien to himself and those about him. He will fear mutual exchange of ideas, keep his ears shut to anything of a threatening or disturbing nature to him omnipotent image, and listen only with that part of himself which meets and suits his own selfish motives. Absorbed as he is in his irrational concept of himself, his perspective of others will be blurred, and thus such transmitted messages as might be of value to him he will see and receive in terms of his own neurotic distortion. As a result, he will not see others about him as individuals in their own rights or as different from himself. Instead he will tend to revolve most of his perceptions around his own way of life and in so doing will subordinate all else to himself.

The emotionally disturbed person visualizes his audience not as it actually presents itself but in terms of his own neurotic needs. Should his audience be admiring and praiseful of him, he will openly accept it and become an attentive and interested listener. However, should it suddenly become critical, questioning or assertive, he immediately topples from his pedestal while his listeners appear as giants.

Whether speaking or listening to others, the neurotic individual does not pause to reflect or ponder a situation, but is quick to express himself with little concern or meaningful purpose. For the most part, his concern is not so much in involving himself in the total communicative experience as it is in the "what" and the "why" of the situation at hand. He is therefore prevented from listening productively, because his rigid and conflicting attitudes blot out more vital and constructive functions of verbal intercourse. The end result is that in the communicative exchange, such a person, feeling little freedom of inner choice, finds that most of his expression takes the form of dogmatic, prejudiced, bitter, cynical, and hopeless ideas and feelings.

The ineffectual listener lacks full identity with himself or others, and for the most part is blocked and inhibited in his capacity to use healthy means of verbalization. In many communicative situations, he becomes inert, confused and rigid as a result of his disturbed state of being. He will not be able to be open with or to listen spontaneously to others, for his egocentricity makes him shun mutual exchange and free self-expression. The result is a devastating fear of intrusion, criticism or questioning and a jealous fear of sharing his thoughts or feelings with others. He will guard his words and his language will be colored by possessiveness and private-ownership.

In the final analysis, the distracted listener becomes an automatic listener who, parrot-like, listens to words and sounds as though they had no connection with thought or meaning. His vanity compels him to enjoy hearing himself talk and he is more interested in the sound effects of his own conversation than in what others have to say. When others are talking, he sifts out only information best suited to his neurotic needs, blotting out and discarding everything else.

Unable to come down to earth or to reach mutual levels of agreement with others, this type of listener finds it difficult to reveal what he is feeling or talking about. He shows little apparent concern for his audience or for directing the listener's reaction to the discussion at hand. Instead his own blind spots and personality difficulties cause him to create a distance between himself and his listeners and so he seeks refuge in those ivory tower levels of his imagination where he can intellectualize, close his ears · to the truth and protect himself against possible threats to his omnipotence.

The rebellious person regards the communicative situation chiefly as an arena for combat and intellectual survival. Only when he has arrived at a healthy state of being, able to accept himself as he is, less compelled toward self-idealization, will his audience become real. He will then become less unrealistic, be more human, sympathetic and a responsible participant in communicative exchange. And once he has done this, he will see his auditors as his equals and will come to have respect for their individual beliefs and wishes. This achieved, the way is open for effective communication to take place.

Listening with 'A Deaf Ear'

None so deaf as those that will not hear—
—MATTHEW HENRY

W E turn now to those listeners who resort to a pseudo deafness to avoid facing the truth and who will often seem to "hear without ears." Here it is the fear of involvement and a feeling of inner conflict which compels the maintenance of a sort of outer facade of don't care attitudes which will give the semblance of inner peace. Such listeners achieve this by simply shutting their ears to any unpleasantness, and hearing only what they feel they should hear. Two examples of this resigned listening are the so-called henpecked husband who switches off his hearing aid and so shuts out the nagging of his complaining wife, and the patient in the psychiatrist's office who closes his ears to the often painfully revealing and truthful interpretations of the therapist.

Driven by his need to avoid struggle and conflicting situations and by his fear of closeness and human involvement, the resigned listener, anxious to settle on the peace-at-any-price basis, accepts his role of onlooker as it pertains to himself and to the world he lives in. The price he pays for this self-imposed restriction—and this he does not realize—is a narrowing of his interests in all vital areas of his life.

In conversation, this same person feels himself constantly threatened. As a result of his imagined fears, he is insecure, defensive, and in need of maintaining a distance between himself and others. Compelled to draw back and retreat into a position of aloofness, he becomes an habitual passive listener and gives very little of himself in the communicative exchange. From time to time, he manifests spurts of aliveness and interest to the extent that he will perhaps offer a few words, but he will at once draw back into his protective shell. This he *must* do because for him participation in any form of life-activity creates an imbalance in his neurotic status quo. That he is driven to protect at all costs.

The resigned person is unable to face himself realistically and his fear of seeing himself as he actually is causes him to repress and deny many of his real feelings, wishes and beliefs. Instead of living fully, he places taboos, checks and inhibitions in the path of his expressions. He is also strongly opposed to putting forth effort or realistic struggle in the attaining of his life goals, for this would mean conscious exertion and that would destroy his carefully erected illusion of peace and tranquillity. He rationalizes his neurotic choice with the belief that life is too short to get excited over or to worry about. So he prefers to minimize or flatly deny his real wishes or potentialities by limiting himself to a form of self-imposed confinement where he is able to keep in balance his neurotic machinery and thus avoid subjecting himself to the necessity for experiencing either pain or struggle.

In order to reinforce his solution, such an individual takes pride in thinking that he can control his environment at will. He feels he can "turn on and off" his hearing to suit his own selfish wishes. By listening only to whatever he feels is not harmful to his protective structures and by disturbing and endangering messages, he believes he can avoid being hurt while at the same time he will give the appearance of being well coordinated. However, what he fails to see is that, at a deeper level, here is a restriction of real desires. For in denying himself participation in struggle and pain, he is also depriving himself in great measure of the awareness of being alive. And, since he must be so compulsively selective in his listening, his communicative exchange is of necessity interfered with and narrowed in its larger scope.

Driven. by his inner dictates, he also is constantly on guard as to the words he permits himself to hear, ever ready to eliminate whatever should be censored and rejected. He is no longer a free agent in making a spontaneous choice. As a result, he will become more and more despairing and exasperated as he is forced to admit that he cannot deny the truth to himself. He will have to face the further realization that it is impossible to exist without some pain, effort or struggle. While his avoidance of real living and his seeking to remain aloof and self-sufficient may give him momentary freedom from anxiety, he will find that he can gain this freedom only by the sacrifice within himself of any true feelings, inspiration or purpose.

In the area of communication, he finds the very intent to speak or to listen objectionable. Because of his own inner restrictions and his reluctance to be one of a group, he feels constantly trapped, coerced and pushed into listening, and will do so only when he feels safe or that it is essential. So he becomes a *partial* listener, one who listens in sections or categories, blotting out the larger areas of perception. Communication then grows strained as the listening exchange becomes rigid, stilted and difficult. He will develop a tendency toward defective feedback relays and his replies will be marked by a cautious holding on to the same words, sounds and phraseology. These responses will be made with little effect and with the use of the fewest possible words. He will employ such phrases by way of retort as: "uh, uh,"—"I see,"—"Anything you say is all right with me,"—"That's all I have to say,"—"There's no need to discuss it further!"

The process of nonparticipation in this form of listening compels this individual to keep in check his true feelings and convictions, resulting in a constant holding back of spontaneous self-expression, a form of rigidity which will prevent him from keeping his ears open to any change to challenge. As a result this fear of change enters into almost every phrase of his life and so he regards his world in general with a pessimistic outlook and judges it as hopeless and unalterable.

As he listens, this type of person will pay very little attention to what is being said, will often seem to be staring right through the speaker. His concentration is notably faulty and scattered and though he may appear to be following the content of the discussion, his thoughts are more than likely to be wandering off in another area. Again because his fear of involvement keeps him at an emotional distance from others, most of his relating is performed either on an intellectual or a mechanical level. He depends largely on his eyes and nose as assists in enabling him to hear and follow what is going on. For this listener the sensory receptors are most important in communicating with others. It can truthfully be said of such people that they have not only deaf ears but deaf hearts.

A person of this make-up rarely gets down to earth in conversations. Instead he speaks from a stratosphere of abstract and hazy words, is seldom humorous, and assumes a pessimistic attitude toward most situations. He does not listen to the essence of the matter under discussion, rarely comprehends with any totality, and mechanically picks at the circumstantial and detailed facts of a discussion point by point. He gives very little of himself as a human being in the exchange, preferring always to use his energies in avoiding the realistic issues and in maintaining his emotional distance. When a discussion gets too close to his feelings, and so is experienced as disturbing to himself, he stuffs cotton in his ears figuratively speaking and pulls out of the situation. He then soars to a high altitude where all verbalization becomes hazy and vague, and he can move into his ivory tower. No longer able to listen or wanting to listen, he will rationalize his actions on the premise that people talk too much nonsense today anyway, that it is too much trouble to listen and get involved, and, that in the long run it really doesn't matter.

Conflicted people will resort to every kind of distraction and protective device when they do not want to listen. They will seem bored or disinterested, and will manage to keep the conversation to a minimum by making the smallest possible contribution to the discussion. Should they find themselves forced to remain in the discussion and listen, they will often psychically remove themselves by becoming sleepy and yawning incessantly, by allowing various objects to distract their attention or by concentrating on activities not directly concerned with the conversation at hand. Or they may attempt to distract their companions and disrupt their trend of thought by coughing, jingling keys or coins, looking at a watch, by deliberately turning on television. The aim throughout all of these devices is to so becloud the listener's own thinking and that of the speaker that, by so keeping their fears at bay, they are able to avoid personal involvement, and thus achieve what is actually a false inner peace.

A person like this is under continual pressure and strain. He rarely feels at ease, or relaxed, but is constantly forced to protect and guard himself against fully experiencing and against communicating his experiences to others. Unable to be spontaneous or to experience a real sense of relatedness with others, he instead develops an all-encompassing hypersensitivity about himself and his relation to those about him. Therefore he is almost always on the defensive in reacting to people.

He avoids taking responsibilities, fears making decisions, and usually waits until the last minute to meet a deadline. In his meetings with others, he listens mostly on the surface, and so receives incoming messages in a muffled state.

142

Most times he camouflages the real issue at hand so as not to be confronted by its true and urgent nature. His own aimlessness and indecisiveness result in difficult areas of distraction which disturb the general trend of the specific listening exchange.

Then too he is given to coloring his responses with a cold detachment, with vague generalizations, intellectualizations and involved elaborations and with confused ideas. He is rarely able to reach communion with his speaker due to that ever-present fear of human contact which of itself disturbs contact with his audience. Because of his hazy abstractions and his inability to come down to earth, this listener will often frustrate his speaker because he will not reveal whether he is listening effectively or whether he is comprehending at least part of what is said. He has little apparent concern for his audience or for establishing emotional rapport with his speaker. Instead he seems to be miles away, speaking from an ivory tower and conveying only a sense of emptiness and ineffectiveness.

When a person such as this feels himself caught and entangled in his neurotic web, he becomes inert and dissatisfied with his way of life, nor will he find satisfaction in his work or in any contact or verbal exchange with others. This imprisoned-like existence makes him think of his own spontaneous desires and expectations as *shoulds* or as impositions coming from the outside. Any necessity for revealing himself either in words or through his gestures or attitudes he regards as coercion to be met with rebellion, passive resistance and inertia. Regarding every form of participation with a sense of strain, he accordingly restricts his activities, including those of speaking and listening, to a minimum. Because of this, he invariably feels constantly frustrated, unhappy, chronically fatigued and unproductive.

A patient of mine who had been in therapy for about six months made most of his responses by means of a monosyllabic yes or no, or with a nod of his head, indicating little self-interest or involvement with his problems. He would block off his hearing so that he had difficulty in listening whenever I got close to his protective defenses, and due to his ever-present fear of anxiety and of going to pieces, he developed numerous resistances to treatment. After many months of slowly developing a relationship which would permit the penetration of his character armor without too severe a pull at his defenses or too strongly disturbing his structure, he began to be less cautious and on the defensive and to permit some messages to reach him. At this time he brought to one of his hours in my office the following dream which poignantly illustrates his struggle against his listening to the truth about himself: "I had some difficulty listening to a far away voice which seemed to come closer to me, booming louder as it came. It frightened me at first. I began pulling at some earwax which offered resistance. I then grasped a tough parasitic worm about five inches long, and slowly drew it out, thereby clearing my ear. But then I became even more frightened. In disgust I quickly dropped the thing, and it suddenly turned into a wriggling centipede. With a piece of newspaper I tried to crush it in order to have the evidence of the experience for the doctor who, I believe, in real life is yourself."

Because this type of individual tends to listen mostly from a distance, so rarely gets to the heart of a situation, and most of his sounds are muffled. In conversation with others, he feels anxieties and so will keep his listening exchange at almost the vanishing point. On the other hand he is likely to feel at ease when alone. Alone, he is able symbolically to carry on conversations with himself without disrupting the protection he must have for his neurotic state. Being introspective, he puts himself apart and above other people, viewing others with superiority, disbelief or disdain, and frequently treating them as if they were objects or things or numbers, never considering himself an integral part of the situation. Since he sees people as nonidentifiable hazy images, he manages to protect himself from involvement by binding his emotional reactions to concepts and ideas rather than to people or things.

In any communicative exchange, the individual with an observer personality is highly gifted in dealing with digital or verbal language, but will tend to neglect analogic, pictorial or nonverbal languages.[1] In other words he thinks and listens in terms of formulae rather than in terms of pictorial images. He listens to *words* rather than *feelings*. Although his capacity for abstractions and theoretical grasping is good, it is in his ability to relate to others as a human being that he is defective.

In an exchange of messages, his need to place everything on an abstract and intellectual level makes it difficult for him to acknowledge the presence of the other person. His defensive and cautious position makes his listening strained and distant, resulting in distractions and a disturbance in his ability to acknowledge the other's message or communicative intent. Therefore it is difficult for him to listen effectively or for him to interpret what others would impart. Also his need to judge most situations with too little feeling of his own rigid points of view create resentment and hostility in his auditors. Whenever he ventures to make a statement, he demands immediate acknowledgment. Yet he will deny others the gratification that he seeks for himself. Actually he increases the confusion even further because he neither explains nor gives any hints as to how his statements ought to be interpreted. And therefore as Ruesch says, "because of his idiosyncratic symbolization system, his minimization of emotions, and his failure to acknowledge others, he is a lonely person who rarely achieves the pleasure of mutual understanding."[2]

Fearing most communicative exchange, he usually manages to separate the meaning of verbal messages from their

145

affective correlations and meanings. Furthermore his abstract thinking and his coldly intellectual and impersonal attitudes toward others cut him off from participating actively in the communicative exchange, and his fear of relating closely to others makes him of necessity only a partial and disinterested listener given to creating static and impersonal barriers between himself and others.

Such a person is extremely sensitive to noise and so, almost as if he were wearing ear muffs, he will automatically close his ears to anything resembling unpleasantness. Although he has a compulsion to translate most feelings into words, he fears and shuns those which might bring him either closer to himself or to others or such as would reveal any of his inner weaknesses or discrepancies. In conversing, he prefers to remain on the periphery of the situation, passively pretending to listen. He wishes only to intellectualize and in that way to arrive at a calculating, definite, abstract solution to any given matter. Because he fears intimacy, he prefers to use a casual conversation as a means for the settling of an issue. He will listen only to his own answers, arrogantly denying to others the same freedom of expression.

From early childhood, this listener has learned to solve his inner contradictions and anxieties by withdrawing from reality and becoming a non-participating spectator in life. He has also discovered—usually painfully—that it is better for him to disinvolve himself from emotional contact with others and instead to objectify his feelings by attentively watching others' actions and ignoring their words. He has thus cut off communicative exchange, and to compensate for this self-induced loneliness and isolation, he prides himself in believing that nothing is so important for him that he cannot do without it. What he does not see is that the very essence of his resignation is a restriction of active desire in all areas of his life and a pervasive absence of goal-direction and planning of his own vital life activities.

Because of this negative approach to the communicative exchange, this person can only produce negative reactions in others. Their failure to acknowledge his desire to communicate only serves to heighten his sense of isolation. His difficulty in responding in a positive vein to others can only create a disturbance in the communicative situation—messages will be improperly relayed and therefore the whole feedback mechanism will become defective. Moreover his fear of eliciting inquiries from his associates will cause him to be overly cautious and defensive when listening, and will therefore contribute to his failure to grasp the total situation.

Because of his habitual resignation, this neurotic will tend to grow introspective. The immobilizing tendency of such a neurotic process acts as a check on initiative, effort, active wishes and strivings—in effect on any natural drive toward self-realization. Both in terms of his idealized and his real self, according to Horney, "he lays an emphasis on *being*, not on *attaining* or *growing*."[3]

Because of the negative and static character of resignation, such a person loses much of his communicative skill and frequently in his inability to relate constructively to others, he will exhibit a lack of aliveness and zest. In conversation he dissociates himself from any personal contact and avoids any mundane or too ordinary subject. He shuns philosophical or weighty discussions. At a given point he retreats into forced silence. If present at any true interchange of words, ideas and feelings, he is the first to remove himself from the situation. Turning off his "earphones," he hastens to escape behind a screen of passivity and rebellious entrenchment. He translates both his hypersensitivity to coercion and his dread of personal involvement into a powerful appeal for *independence* and *freedom*, his argument being that it is natural for man to want freedom, and that he must not, as a human being, feel forced to listen against his will to any one or anything.

147

However as we look at some of his arguments and examine them, we find that this idea of freedom is a negative one since it implies a freedom *from* rather than *for* himself.

In listening to others, this same person does not select or discriminate properly. He misuses new information; he does not learn from disagreements; and he is unable to reach levels of agreement. In the face of contradictory or conflicting situations, he becomes overwhelmed with anxiety, fears open discussion, and retreats into a shell of silent resistance. In his need for clear cut dichotomies, he goes all out for one side of any issue, completely ignoring the other. Confronted with evidence of his prejudiced and dogmatic viewpoint, he becomes so firmly entrenched in his negative position that it is increasingly difficult to dissuade him from his premature decisions and impulsive actions. Thrown into open contact with others, he recoils from fighting by withdrawing from the battlefield and declaring himself uninterested.

When the listening becomes difficult for him to understand or requires added mental exertion, he will refuse to face up to the task, rationalizing his action on the basis that living with others is difficult enough in any case and there is little purpose or use in putting increased effort into making a go of it. Most of us are guilty daily of doing just this. If we are not able immediately to comprehend what some one is trying to tell us or if a topic for discussion becomes a bit too difficult, we avoid listening to it by appearing to be tired or confused or vague. If what a radio or television speaker is saying is too involved or lengthy, we turn him off and look for a less taxing program—anything just so we don't have to search within ourselves for the resources required in serious thinking. We prefer to remain on the periphery of our conscious selves involved only superficially rather than to face up to a situation which may make demands on our intellects. Just so does the disinterested listener fears making real effort when listening and so he seeks easier and easier listening. Generally speaking he listens only to such things as are simplified and handed to him on a platter, choosing to avoid any planned or periodic effort necessary to listen to difficult material. Another rationalization he uses for not concentrating when listening is that most situations are uninteresting and dull to begin with, and have been encountered so often that there is no point in being concerned over them. In this way he finds a suitable excuse for his inability to involve himself personally in the discussion or to give of himself honestly in the communicative exchange. As G. K. Chesterton once said, "there is no such thing as an uninteresting subject; there are only uninterested people."

Our neurotic fears disagreement at all costs and as a defense against this he will prematurely refuse listening to any controversial subject on the grounds that it is uninteresting. With a wave of his hand, he places himself above involving himself in differences or arguments— another of his rationalizations for not listening.

Cicero once cried aloud, "For God's sake, disagree with me, so that there can be two of us!" Like Cicero, most of us believe that differences in opinion and concept do make for aliveness and lead by direct line to an active verbal exchange. However there are always those who will resort to idle and wasteful argument to avoid facing real issues. They are neither interested in nor desirous of hearing what others have to say nor in having others listen to them.

Listening with inclination and with open ears should be instrumental in giving an air of freedom to the flow of any communicative exchange, particularly if both speaker and listener share a sense of mutuality, flexibility, and understanding. Such an awareness will be of tremendous value in preventing a conversation from reaching an impasse, an experience common to resigned listeners.

The more resigned a person is, the more psychically paralyzed, hopeless and dissatisfied he will feel about himself and his way of life. And in his relation to others, the greater his sense of withdrawal, the less will he be able to communicate effectively and the more distractions and disturbances will be present in the path of his listening. Only as he becomes less alienated and immobilized will he begin to discover his real self and want to participate more actively and realistically with his surroundings. By so doing, he will become more of a complete and functioning human being and so a more productive listener in the communicative situation.

References

1, 2. Jurgen Ruesch: *Disturbed Communication.* New York, Norton & Company, 1957, pp. 130-133.
3. Karen Horney: *Neurosis and Human Growth.* New York, Norton & Company, 1954, p. 272.

Listening with the Third Ear

*To be human is to speak. To be abundantly human is
to speak freely and fully. The converse of this is a profound
truth, also: that the good listener is the best physician for
those who are ill in thought and feeling.*

—WENDELL JOHNSON

An understanding of and feeling for what goes on when
one person talks and another listens is the foundation stone
for modern techniques in the practice of psychotherapy.
Disturbances in communication when properly evaluated
are considered as distortions either in perception (listening)
or in transmission (speaking). Therefore most important
as a corrective agent in personality disturbances is the
communicative interaction between patient and therapist.

Psychotherapy might perhaps best be defined as an
effort at improving the ability of the patient to communicate within himself and with others. Modern therapy
stresses the treatment of the *total* personality, the *whole*
man, and is directed toward a reorientation of the individual's relation to himself (intrapersonal network) as
well as toward his disturbances in relation to others (interpersonal network). Its main emphasis is in understanding
such disturbances of communication as are present, that
to be followed by the correction of the defective processes.
It also tends to lead the individual out of his neurotic
development by making available to him whatever resources are possible toward healthy growth. The more
such a person is helped and directed toward liberating
the forces of spontaneous growth, the more awareness,

151

understanding, and sense of being will he have for himself. Hence the ideal in any worthwhile psychotherapeutic approach is the liberation and utilization of those energies and forces which may lead to effective communication and to self-realization.

Psychoanalysis has taught us to grasp the deep significance of the relationship between word and action. In the early days, the psychotherapist functioned more as a mirror in which the patient saw his moods, thoughts and feelings reflected. In a conscious effort to maintain himself in a wholly objective fashion and fearing to involve himself with his patient, the therapist was so preoccupied with the *why* that he revealed very little of himself as a human being. Because he used few words and communicated through intellectual verbal pathways which used silence as a vehicle of control, he blocked many of the possibilities for real contact.

Today the therapist presents himself and communicates with his patient on a more interpersonal basis. With his "third ear," he listens not only to the words his patient speaks but also to his (the therapist's) own "inner voice," and to what emerges therefrom. At all times, he strives to communicate with and feel a real interest in his patient, to see him as a suffering entity and to reach within him for what is basically growing and resourceful.

In an effective psychotherapy process, the therapist must be keen and alert enough to look behind the patient's contrived screen of verbalizations nor must he be taken in by the disguising maneuver of this talkativeness. It is essential for him to keep in mind that there is meaning in whatever his patient says, in his gestures, movements, tensions, pauses or silences, in his reflections, mannerisms, muscular reactions and a score of other communing factors. Listening to the words as words only may be most deceiving.

In this patient-therapist relationship, many first impressions and instinctive reactions are communicated either

152

directly or non-directly through both verbal and non-verbal channels. Therefore the *psychotherapist's most important tool is listening*. If his listening posts are perceptive enough, he will gain valuable information through the tone of a patient's voice, its many inflections and nuances, his choice of words, the rhythm and tempo of his speech and so on.

An astute therapist early in his career will train himself to listen and observe with his fullest concentration and comprehension to what is presented both in the form of direct literal verbal content and in the many subterfuges and deep hidden emotions, repressed thoughts and symbolic expressions which go on beneath the more obvious levels of awareness.

It is said that the therapist, like his patient, often knows things without knowing that he knows them. It has been said that "the voice that speaks in him, speaks low, but he who listens with a third ear hears also what is expressed almost noiselessly, what is said *pianissimo*."[1]

For instance, there are times in psychoanalysis when the statements made by a patient are not consciously heard by the analyst, yet they are understood and interpreted. The therapist who allows information to flow passively through his ears without immediately examining every aspect and using his selective powers in the discrimination or scrutiny of what is before him, may very well lose the psychological moment for seizing elusive material. Here—and only here—as Reik says, "you must leap before you look; otherwise you will be looking at a void where a second before a valuable impression flew past."[2]

The *third ear* is what Freud referred to when he said the capacity of the unconscious for fine hearing was one of the requisites for the psychoanalyst. It can be turned inward so as to hear voices within the self that are otherwise not audible because they are drowned out by the noise of conscious thought-processes. In the practice of psychoanalysis, it is well for the therapist to listen to this inner voice with more attention than to what "reason" tells about the unconscious. He must also be acutely aware of what is said inside himself, *écouter aux voix intérieures*, and "shut his ear to the noises of adult wisdom, well-considered opinion, conscious judgment."

It is essential that the therapist at all times be sensitive to, listen, understand and recognize the secret meanings of the imperceptible and personal character of the language the patient uses. And so that he may receive, record, and decode the patient's impressions successfully, he must listen productively without criticism, prejudice or condemnation, and he must also assimilate this information. Only when he has formed a total picture of his patient's verbal and non-verbal symbols in terms of his own impressions, will the therapist be able to arrive at an honest evaluation of the issues at hand.

The Role of Listening in the Therapeutic Process

The first section of the therapeutic process takes place primarily on the conscious or verbal level. The patient speaks; we gather together pertinent data and we ask leading questions. As the patient continues to communicate in speech or is silent, we listen attentively and follow each of his gestures, peculiarities, bodily manifestations or presenting movements, all of which communicate some vital expression of his actions, feelings, beliefs and tensions.

The next step requires more concentrated and selective hearing. It consists in listening to psychological data, deciphering its hidden messages, assimilating most of its contents, and then in attempting to activate our own selves as we communicate in relative exchange with the patient.

Once the preliminary interviews are over, the therapist may tell his patient something of the therapeutic process to be undertaken. He then will suggest that the patient relax and allow himself to say whatever occurs to him— *just as he sees, feels and experiences it*—in his own word concepts. Since at this point listening of a more sensitive and higher caliber is needed, the third ear now goes into action. At this point, the therapist must attune himself not only to what may appear on the surface but to all hidden emotions and thoughts both in his patient and in himself. He must become a *silent observer* who listens to the words and their impulses as they come from the patient's verbal and non-verbal language, and searches within himself the while for the means to direct and promote mutual growth in this newly established relationship.

In the initial visits, it may be better for the therapist to listen in relative silence. At first the patient may understandably be alarmed by this move. Yet he will soon come to welcome it as something which calms him and gives him a chance to speak freely and at his own tempo without fear of the conventional inhibitions and interruptions. He will also come to feel that his therapist, through his silent and reflective listening, is giving him, the patient, the fullest benefit of his attention, interest and sympathy. In such an atmosphere of mutal acceptance and understanding is created the solid basis for the transference relationship.

One of the best means of self-expression in psychotherapy is obtained through the use of free-associations. Through this communicative channel, the patient is usually helped to relax, to feel free to speak spontaneously, and to move as far as possible away from conventional everyday adaptations. In this process, the patient in pouring out a spate of words, unconsciously reveals things about himself which, had he been aware of their relatedness, he might have kept back. If the therapist is actively listening for slips of the tongue, word distortions, accidental gestures or expressions or other psychological cues, he should be able to help his patient realize that above and beyond his obvious verbal productions he is either retaining or resisting his awareness of some other more hidden and painful material. And if the patient shows through words, vocal sounds or similar signals that he has understood this, then some connection, understanding and working through of the problems will have begun.

There are times when, due to a novice therapist's eagerness for interpretations, he will want to move in compulsively and talk instead of just listening. In compulsive neurotics to whom talkativeness is a powerful tool, an attempt at being rational and arguing a patient's problems out has been known to prove most devastating. With this kind of a patient, the silent passive attitude in the beginning phases of treatment gives him something he has never before received—a serious and sympathetic interest in his irrational fears and symptoms.

In communicating with his patient, the therapist will best help him if he listens attentively to and, in turns, uses the language best understood by the patient. To use standard psychoanalytic jargon and cliches will too frequently confuse and misdirect the therapeutic process. The more experienced therapist is one who hears and communicates in words and who also sees, feels and senses the total participation of his patient in conflict.

In the final process of growth, *the last word, to repeat, must belong to the patient.* For the most part, the patient can and will change if and when he understands the reasons why he should do so. By helping the patient to be silent at times and listen to his own inner voice, the therapist directs him toward putting his own conflicts and inner tensions into words, thereby removing those obstacles which interfered with emotional growth by permitting him to free his verbalizations from hindering contradictions and confusions. In good time this will effect a release of the patient's grip on his neurotic entanglements.

The Therapist as a Listener

In order to function at some level of competency and listen effectively to others, the therapist should have most or some of the following essential requirements:

(1) he should have his own personal problems reasonably worked through or at least be so aware of them that they will not interfere with his relating constructively with others;

(2) he must have an inherent belief in man's ability to change and grow toward self-realization, and a feeling for process in changing, a knowledge of the patient's fear of it, and the skill to handle defenses against it effectively;

(3) he must in every aspect of his personality himself be a human being, with a sympathy for those who struggle and suffer, and the wish to use every human attribute within himself toward expressing warmth, understanding, sincerity, and respect for the patient's own wishes and rights. Once the patient has discovered this feeling of mutuality and shared understanding with his therapist, he will have won half the battle;

(4) finally, he must to some degree be trained and well oriented in the dynamics of the neurosis. He must be practiced in the art of good listening and flexible enough to use as many therapeutic tools as will help toward effecting change; he must alert his hearing to all available healing forces in the patient and start mobilizing these constructive assets right at the very onset of the therapy. He should also be able and confident enough to handle most eventualities that may occur in the therapeutic situation and be himself integrated enough to "listen between the lines," so as to assimilate them without too destructive counterreactions. To this end, he must handle his own anxieties and hostilities without harming the patient's progress at the time.

Disturbed Listening Posts in Therapy

Successful communication is only possible when the participants' moods are attuned to each other on an equal level of feeling and affection. To facilitate this interaction the therapist must present himself as a good listener so that he can become truly understanding and wholly sincere with his patients.

Often when an individual seems anxious or in distress, he really doesn't want advice. What he is actually looking for is someone to talk to freely, someone who will at the same time make no evaluative judgments but rather will slowly direct him to the discovery of his own inner resources. In the final analysis, what the patient wants is to free himself of his neurotic shackles so that he may become a responsible and resourceful person, capable of making use of his own constructive energies. Then he will have started on the road toward self-realization.

It is not easy to listen to someone else's ideas, thoughts and feelings effectively. The so-called verbose type, for instance, will disturb true communication by distorting issues, and by attempting to place his conflicts, feelings and hidden motivations on an intellectual level. He takes pride in his wisdom and intellect. He thinks for the most part in absolutes, and many of his responses are purely rational. His own inner fear of his feelings compels him always to seek for logical and clean-cut answers to his problems.

For such patients, words act as a defense against action. For these, "speaking" means "doing," and so they believe that verbalizing can relieve them from real activity. They have or feel little responsibility for what they say, and their word diarrhea represents a neurotic attempt at solution and a discharge of tension. There are some people who fear seeing into themselves who will talk and talk without actually saying anything. On this, Meerloo writes: "the multitude of words and associations is used to disguise the process of revelation of what is really hidden. In their logorrhea they want to pin down the analyst, to hurt his ears, to make him confused—all this in order not to track the important subjects."[3]

The therapist must be constantly on the alert not to be narcotized by words. If his listening posts are not attuned properly, he will easily become the victim of such an outpouring of words.

What is basically essential in any therapist-patient relationship is a feeling of cooperation, flexibility, honesty and mutual growth. Both collaborators should have their listening posts attuned to such a degree of selectivity that they can participate in what for both of them is a creative atmosphere of give-and-take. Neither individual need necessarily feel himself the superior; neither should be viewed as more important than the other, nor should either participant have to deny or eliminate himself. In such a spirit of teamwork, according to Wassell, "each according to his ability and availability, a solid doctor-patient relationship can be established which will help the patient to face, experience, understand and eventually resolve his inner dividedness, so that he can emerge a free and distinct individual."[4]

Disturbances in the therapeutic relationship also arise as a result of difficulties within the therapist himself. The presenting character structure of the therapist, with all of its neurotic residuals, tends to inhibit, block and retard movement in any particular therapeutic process. A strict intellectual approach, for instance, or any illusion of superiority blocks the therapist's own self-growth and consequently hinders his working effectively with his patients. In our particular society today, many view the therapist as some sort of a god-like magician or master mind who is capable of knowing all and solving all the problems of the world. This pride in intellect and know-all attitude is further supported by the mass media of

159

television, movies, magazine articles and novels where the therapist is usually depicted as a robot-like thinking machine, a sort of push-button which automatically simplifies, through his use of words, most of the complexities of our day. As a result, he becomes shrouded with a mantle of mysterious wisdom and is placed on an ivory-tower level where he can be seen, heard, but not touched.

The following are some of the types of therapists that I would like to categorize as being ineffectual listeners:

1. THE ANXIOUS OVER-TALKATIVE THERAPIST

This is usually the therapist who, because of his own inner needs to succeed and achieve results in his work with others, is too eager to get ahead or to control and influence his patients. He uses words to persuade, encourage, mould, coerce or plead. He will insist upon and stress the speeding up the tempo of the analysis in order to go full force ahead, to plunge into problems, and so he will over-encourage struggle. He will anververbalize in his work, rarely listen, be fearful of silences, and be too anxious to ask leading and razor-like questions, in the hope that the answers he receives will suit his own egocentric demands for adapting his patient to his own concepts of living. In more desperate moments, if frustrated as to the results in his therapy, he may resort to using his *therapeutic immunity* as a weapon to strike back at his patients. What may then ensue is that either the patient becomes so frightened of this approach that he feels compelled to terminate treatment or his feeling of resentment toward the therapist becomes so intense that, for fear of retaliation, he will repress his true feelings and remain passively angered. In both instances, however, while the therapeutic relationship may assume the appearance of much going on, little real rapport exists and hence little change takes place in the patient.

160

2. The "So-called" Silent Therapist

In this group we find the therapist who, because of his own fear of involvement or intrusion, conducts over-cautiously and, unable to tackle a problem directly, is fearful of struggle and anxiety. His hands-off policy and his need for utter privacy compel him to remain aloof and at a distance from his patient in an effort to keep things at status quo. Should the patient in turn express a wish or desire for warmth, friendliness or closeness, such a therapist may immediately become anxious and interpret this as an attempt by the patient to become too personal. He furthers estrangement in communication by wording most of his interpretations or comments in a language of objectivity and therapeutic jargon, with little feeling for its actual human connotations. He likes to coin new phrases, to have pet theories of his own, and, parrot-like, to seduce his patients so that they will introduce into their own vocabularies these very phrases which will then be vicariously experienced by himself. Such a therapist may feel that by saying too much about himself or by expressing his feelings about his patients he will disturb or inflate them, thereby furthering the degree of impersonality, and the whole purpose of communication as an area of spontaneity and mutual exchange of feelings, ideas and beliefs becomes thwarted. The therapeutic situation will tend to become over-objectivized, over-intellectualized, cold at the periphery, and in a rut. Whatever the neurotic residuals present in a greater or lesser degree in the therapist, they of necessity will interfere with and block the degree of change and movement in the therapeutic work. It is my own conviction that no therapist can do other than present and show himself as a human being in any given relationship. If, instead, he chooses to act the role of the popular conception, i.e. the detached analyst sitting beyond the couch in his ivory-tower abode, then the therapeutic situation—of necessity—takes on an aura of intellectual curiosity, cold detachment and becomes mechanical in form.

3. The Soothing Therapist

Finally we have a third kind of therapist who, because of his own sense of compliancy and a need for unobtrusiveness, tends to bend over backwards and to place too much stress in pleasing his patient and putting him at constant ease. He likes to give the impression of listening to almost everything. For fear of keeping his patients at too great a distance and because of his own fear of being unaccepted, rebuffed or rejected, he may tend to move in immediately, to show attitudes of over-friendliness, chumminess, sacrifice and, in some cases, over-protectiveness. Because of his own aversion to anxiety or struggle, he may feel constantly compelled to make his patients comfortable, to avoid permitting them to remain in conflict for too long a time. He further tends to foster the belief that any open demonstration of irritability, anger or resentment is to be avoided and denied at all costs. This is a fallacious approach because, while the constructive expression of such feelings in a patient—for instance, in one who fears expressing anger toward others—may prove shocking and difficult to accept at first, once he feels that it is acceptable to others, he may risk similar feelings with himself. I believe that any action on the part of the therapist that promotes activity and an alive motion in the therapeutic situation should be communicated to the patient. It is here that the useful selection of verbal or non-verbal material with its proper timing and method of communication is of utmost importance.

The Road toward Inner Freedom

In the final analysis, the therapist's main goal is to foster mental health and growth in his patients. In this process of maturation, he of course must keep in mind that growth is never progressively pure, that it involves relativistic values and more or less proportions. Within this framework, mental health may be defined as one's ability to communicate healthily to one's self, to others, and to one's social structure as a whole. The network of communication depends for its success not so much on its nature as on its relative ability to withstand temporary breakdowns as experienced in tensions, frustrations, somatic complaints, etc., and on the resourcefulness of its inner machinery to reestablish lines of communications, thus repairing areas of maladjustment and disorganization.

The therapist who best serves his patient's needs is the one who listens to the fullest of his capacities—condensing, abstracting and decoding as he goes along, always being careful lest he interrupt the already established communicative system of interrelatedness. At the same time he will attempt to be most selective in his listening and in his choice of words, so that he may arrive at the best available conclusions and yet not appear too artificial.

In beginning the therapy, it is essential to select carefully and mobilize all constructive and resourceful assets present in the patient. Later on, as the patient moves away from the surface of his conflicts and begins to get closer to himself, he will have less of an oblivious reaction to his remoteness from himself and more of an awareness and interest concerning his real feelings, wishes and beliefs. During this period, it is of the utmost importance that the therapist listen effectively.

As his alienation fades the patient will be more absorbed in the questions "Who am I?" and "What do I want?", etc., and it is imperative that the analyst be there to decode this message. With his growing sensitivity, the patient will now begin to question many of his existing attitudes, feelings and beliefs, and to re-evaluate them in the light of reality and of his own inner volition and beginning independence.

The road toward inner freedom begins as the patient feels himself on more solid ground and more capable of grappling with and facing his conflicts. In so doing, he will tend less to project and rationalize his problems on the outside, experiencing them instead as coming from somewhere within himself. At long last, he will see himself less as a god-like image and he will acquire an earnest desire to develop his own given potentials as a human being.

When the battle toward self-realization is finally won, great constructive forces become available to the patient. He will now have reached the level where he can assume more responsibility for directing his own way of life; and will be ready to give up many of his fictitious values and so to discard his illusions about himself. Accordingly as he moves closer to himself, he will have acquired a basic change in his concept of values, a new way of life and more realistic goals.

In the end process of therapy, however, the inner communicating systems of insight must function before any real or lasting change can ensue. Acceptance by ear or intellect of one's conflicts without bodily participation or true awareness will give but temporary relief and will produce in the long run merely a verbal expression of self. One must become wholly aware of his own conflicts in feeling and conscious knowledge before lasting and effective integration can take place.

When this stage has been reached, the patient will be able to listen to what goes on at the very core of his being and inner consciousness. He will direct his attention and concentration to those levels within himself where he can reflect about the world about him and communicate with his true feelings, beliefs and desires. His playback mechanism will have become so adaptive that it will permit him to become realistically perceptive and selective in his listening, and to choose in terms of *what is* rather than of *what should be*. This will give him greater spontaneity in flexibility, confidence and multi-valued concepts.

In conclusion, the more a person knows himself, the more effectively will he be able to listen and to communicate with himself and to others. In addition he will have greater courage and confidence in accepting himself and others in their true perspectives. He will have freed himself of many of his prejudices, irrational fears, inhibitions and imaginative magic ideals. In this process of growing, he will be ready to face realities with his existing resources, to listen to the truth of the matter, to accept himself as he is with all of his shortcomings, and, finally, to recognize himself as an integral part of the world in which he lives.

References

1, 2. Theodor Reik: *Listening with The Third Ear*. New York, Farrar-Straus and Company, 1949, p. 145.
3. Joost A. M. Meerloo: *Conversation and Communication*. New York, International Universities Press, Inc., 1952, p. 218.
4. Benjamin Wassell: "The Analytic Relationship." *The American Journal of Psychoanalysis*, Vol. XV, No. 1, 1955.

The Sound of Silence

Every sound shall end in silence, but the silence never dies.
—SAMUEL MILLER HOGEMAN

W E have a magnificent ability for not listening and remaining silent whenever we don't or won't listen to something. For instance, as one of a large group of people we often converse with but one or two and are yet able to block out the surrounding din. Schilder refers to experiments showing that when the third temporal convolution of the brain was anesthetized, subjects complained of hearing too many spontaneous sounds. This work suggests the possibility of central suppressor areas which protect our being overwhelmed by noise. Only with the aid of these, as Knapp once said, can the "sense of hearing be at once so acute and so selective. Otherwise we would live in bedlam."

Auditory and visual stimuli come to us in a constant flow from the outside world. Auditory impressions, unlike visual ones, are likely to be more acutely perceptible when we are quiet or asleep. "The day has eyes; the night has ears." But unlike the eyes, the ears are never shut. However, if it were not for the function of auditory repression, sleeping would be impossible if we were to listen to all the sounds that reach our ears. Falling asleep may be characterized as the sudden obliteration of sound and the deepening sense of silence which prevails, just as sudden awareness of sound may signalize awakening—often with a start.

In spite of this awareness, acoustic stimuli and impulses may penetrate into the sleeping state with a persistent yet imperceptible quality. Electroencephalographically it can be shown that, before a sound is loud enough to awaken a person fully, it may affect his brain waves, moving them to a higher level of sleep. This may be one explanation for a mother's particular alertness to her baby's cry or the sleeping soldier's to a warning attack or the fireman's to the clang of the firebell.

On the other hand, we slumber and dream in relative silence. For the most part our dreams are soundless, though occasionally exogenous sounds penetrate into our dreaming activity, causing us to awaken. Dreams, so Knapp colorfully describes them, "resemble silent movies. Scenes change, animation occurs, but seldom are there sharp sensory impressions, particularly acoustic ones. Communication takes place, but we do not often hear the voices of dream figures."[1] In an analysis of over three hundred dreams of six patients under intensive observation, clear sound percepts were reported in only six per cent of these dreams; and with still other patients, the range varied from zero to fourteen per cent.

Actual living occurs primarily on our silent object levels. Whatever we "think," "feel," "believe," or "do" starts silently. Only as a secondary choice does talk begin. In educational procedures, for example, we train our students to be silent and to observe what is going on so that they may evaluate their observations in their true perspective. Silence allows us to use our capacities to the fullest and thus gives the greatest opportunity for observation. The art of silence gives time to look first before speaking, to search deeply within ourselves, to reflect seriously and thus to develop a true creative outlook.

Too many of us are overeager to talk and to make statements on matters which may be foreign to our experience or knowledge. We are too ready to take and accept passively what we hear from others and to regard what we accept as truth without first giving it full expression and experience within ourselves. We become intoxicated with the sound of our own words and make sounds and noises as though they were vibrating from an "empty barrel." The encouragement and use of silence within ourselves will help greatly in lessening this unnecessary communicative evil of superficiality and emptiness, and hopefully will lead to a more effective and purposeful way of self-expression. Productive or reflective silence is a quality which all of us should encourage and develop within ourselves.

In her book *Gift from the Sea*, Anne Morrow Lindbergh has in simple poetic language set forth her definition of that inner peace and serenity which obtains when we have learned to enter into such a state of inner communion with ourselves. She writes:

> Here on this island I have space . . . . Here there is time; time to be quiet; time to work without pressure; time to think; time to watch the heron . . . . Time to look at the stars or study a shell; time to see friends; to gossip, to laugh, to talk. Time, even, *not* to talk . . . . Here on this island I find I can sit with a friend without talking, sharing the day's last sliver of pale green light on the horizon, or the whorls in a small white shell, or the dark scar left in a dazzling night sky by a shooting star. The communication becomes communion and one is nourished as one never is by words.[2]

In our particular society today, whether to talk or to keep quiet is a most perplexing choice. Silence—to many of us—is frightening and something to be avoided at all costs, while the urge to talk for talk's sake is a familiar compulsion. Often we talk simply for the sake of hearing ourselves. As a means of relating to our fellow men, we engage in all sorts of verbal pronouncements and discussions about anything and everything. Too often we fear being silent and to avoid so being we struggle within ourselves to be continually lively and sparkling in our verbal expressions.

The "togetherness" of social contact and the compulsion to talk therefore become the primary factors in conversation while the content of the subject matter is secondary. We come together mainly through our words and not through our feelings. Our daily conversations, our small talk, chit chat, gossip and so on, have given us an important medium of social communication with which to break through the barriers of strangeness and establish between ourselves some form of interrelatedness.

Silence is golden, yet the silent person among us is usually considered as a "quiet type"—a bore. Of keeping quiet, Doctor Crane once wrote in his daily newspaper column, "we muff many golden opportunities to gladden the lonely hearts and inflate the ego of deserving folks who are discouraged by lack of friendly praise. . . . God expects all Christians to be good salesmen. And salesmen are not noted for being tongue-tied."

Charles Evans Hughes is reported to have lost the Presidency of the United States because of something he did not say. On a visit to California, Hughes failed to extend friendly overtures to Senator Hiram Johnson who controlled that state politically. It is now said that by his reticence Mr. Hughes so offended and slighted Senator Johnson that the latter threw the state's electoral votes to Woodrow Wilson. The moral of this story could very well be, in view of the evidence at hand, "don't make a fetish of being a silent person."

Silence can also be disturbing in many of our everyday relationships. Our necessity for working with others, the constant contacts with strangers and the accentuation of group life has made talking an essential part of our living. To remain silent in the presence of others may well lead to tension and discord, since an unwillingness to converse is often interpreted as an attitude of unfriendliness.

169

In order to be silent as we listen quietly and perceptively to our inner selves, we must attempt to be concerned chiefly with ourselves and our surroundings. This state of holistic experiencing in itself necessitates the use of not only our sense of hearing, but of the other senses—smell, touch, sight and taste. The blind young Indian, Ved Mehta, in his book *Face to Face*, describes how in a moment of panic as fires were approaching his home and dazed by the preceding days of apprehensive fear, he stopped listening: "There was nothing different to hear, no different smells, and I sensed nothing. My breathing steadied, and my heart stopped throbbing. Was it resignation? Or was it that too much had happened to sort out?" [4]

The opposite of creative silence is silent retreat. The less involved a person is with himself, the more remote he becomes and the less his feelings and surroundings are experienced. Concomitantly, the more abstract his thinking and speaking become, the less he will know himself as an alive human being, the closer he is to becoming an automaton or *thinking machine*.

The further away we move from reality and drift into a world of infinite abstractions, intellectualizations and rationalizations, the more we need our illusions, the more our language becomes superficial, empty, rigid and colored with magical connotations. We develop deep feelings of emptiness and nothingness which in turn become basic sources from which spring increasing hopelessness, resignation and anxiety.

Some of us, when conflicted, feel coerced and pressured in conversation and tend to minimize and shorten our verbal contacts. We are likely to listen passively and to say little, even though we may already have formed opinions. Should a situation arise in which we are actually desirous of expressing ourselves openly, we may instead become rebellious, feel attacked and assume defensive attitudes. So we wait in silent defiance, protesting word-lessly. In so doing, we attempt to rise above the struggle by escaping into our imaginations where we create a false picture of *individuality* and *freedom*. Actually we try to avoid open conflict, defend the *status quo*. This "silent type" idealization of one's self is only one manifestation of a neurotic grandiose self.

The dread of nothingness, if not too vivid, may come to the surface as frantic activity: i.e., compulsive talking, eating and drinking, gay parties, promiscuity, marihuana jags, and even that form of blind destructiveness we know as suicide.

In social groups we are given to the use of what I shall call 'blab' and long circumstantial stories for the purpose of avoiding silence and making conversation. This "blab-itis" serves to hide our innermost thoughts and wishes from ourselves and from others by creating a wall of words between us and our listener. Essentially, by resorting to blab, we keep our listeners at a distance while we bombard and bore them to death with our verbal sounds and noises. In effect we are assuring ourselves that as long as we keep talking, nothing can happen to us and thus we cannot be hurt. This method also serves to protect us, we tend to believe, against the inner voice of our conscience. Little do we know that the impact of this inner communicating force reaches its own natural level of expression and, if thwarted, it will seek more dangerous channels such as emotional depression, psychosomatic illness or other psychic disturbances.

People today are driven by an almost irresistible urge to talk when they get together. In any social group they feel compelled to say something on practically every subject—the weather, their children and relatives, gossip about others, their troubles. To remain silent might easily be interpreted as impolite, unkind or arrogant. Too often we feel attacked by these conversational needs

171

and must defend ourselves against such a threat. It is to avoid this vacuum without words that we use such expressions as "how are you?," "you look well today," "nice day," "goodbye,"—expressions indicative of a relationship or contact with another person—an extension of togetherness. This wish for collective affection through logic and words serves not only to fill the voids of silence, but gives us comfort and a sense of group belonging.

Too many of us use words in a compulsive and empty way, with little feeling for or connection with what we mean to express. Conversation has become an arena for oratorical self-glorification. The more one says, the louder one talks, the more persuasive a speaker one is, the better a success he becomes in most present-day social groups. Repeatedly we refer to the same topics and use the same phraseology in our efforts to avoid a lull in conversation. Pauses and moments of silent meditation disturb us. We are eager to keep up a never-flagging flow of discussion, to race on with the sound of words, to keep words popping constantly. Regard for others, communion with our listeners, or a sense of silent reflection and self-appraisal have become secondary motives.

In talking to each other with better understanding, it is essential that at times *we keep silent*. Today many of us live on the surface because of our *fear of becoming silent* and of having to listen to the truth of the matter. This fear and this lack of inner communion come about as we move away from the core of our true inner feelings and resort to superficial logic and compulsive verbalization.

In avoiding silence, we place a barrage of words between ourselves and any true awareness of reality. We camouflage the true perception of things with falsities and built-up notions and illusions. On the other hand, by becoming silent and searching *actively* and constructively within ourselves for the truth about our actual limitations as well as our real potentialities, we shall arrive at a realistic, dynamic and complete awareness of *what is*, and so shall enter into a truthful and healthy pattern of existence.

In silent meditation we necessarily meet with and experience struggle and conflict, both an inevitable part of living. Conversely, the fear of facing ourselves realistically and the compelling need to be conflict-free, to achieve peace and serenity, can only lead ultimately to further distortions, fears and anxieties. And the use of "rose-colored glasses" in the face of everyday conflicting actualities creates further confusion, self-destructiveness and wasteful living. Only in the experiencing of and the ability to live with everyday struggle and conflict and to accept misery, pain and suffering as an integral part of living do we find a true and positive way of life.

In every true interchange of words and ideas, we must attempt to remove those dogmatic barriers which interfere with inner freedom and flexibility of self-expression. We as a people are too impregnated and influenced with official dogma, social taboos, verbal rigidities and authoritative standard evaluations. We are educated and encouraged to believe more in the judgments and conclusions of so-called wiser and more influential persons than in our own creative intuitions.

In order to promote inner growth and healthy relatedness, we must develop the capacity and the desire to examine ourselves critically, to understand and to reshape our values, attitudes and beliefs. In so doing, we must have the courage to remain silent so that we can listen patiently to our fullest capacity, without prejudice, condemnation or preconceived judgments. Once we approximate this level, we may then be able to experience and perceive the *real truth of the matter* as *it is*.

In the attempt to understand and know ourselves better, we too often either refuse or do not know how to be silent or how to listen effectively. In seeking to understand the true communications within one's self, one must be able to probe deep into one's inner conscience. At these times, it is not enough just to listen to what is said openly. One must also decode the subtle impressions these communications make upon our total being, upon the fleeting thoughts and feelings aroused in the particular communicative experience. In short, the most productive way of penetrating into our secret minds is by remaining silent and by listening holistically. In that way we shall gain a better understanding of ourselves and thus stimulate a vital interest and an active curiosity about ourselves and the surrounding world.

Listening to oneself is difficult because of man's increasing aversion to being alone with himself. Many of us think of a quiet evening at home or an hour or so devoted to quiet reflection as something to be avoided at all cost, a waste of time and an admission of weakness. For some of us, the fear of being alone and silent is so intense that any activity, regardless of its value or purpose, is preferable. As long as we continue to fear facing ourselves, we shall miss the opportunity for listening to ourselves and shall therefore not benefit from the rewards of silent meditation.

Being alone with oneself and remaining silent is often thought of as loneliness. Speech is civilization, silence isolates, so we have been led to believe. Unhappily it is true that modern man is unable to be alone with himself for too long a period of time. Society is moving so fast nowadays that to pause and reflect is often misconstrued as falling behind the times. Our uppermost aim is action; inactivity or silence is frowned upon.

Constantly exposed to the sounds and noise of opinions and ideas which come flowing in from the outside, we have developed a phobia against being alone with our innermost thoughts, feelings, wishes or desires. For the most part we live vicariously through others, denying the truth to ourselves, as we refuse to be silent and listen to the voice of our conscience. It is primarily because of this that the irrational fears of death and of growing old are two of the most common expressions of anxiety today. These fears, which result primarily from the failure to live productively, become accentuated when we are confronted with the stark reality of our inner sense of nothingness and progressive self-deterioration. These irrational fears and ideas are fostered in our society by our emphasis, as Fromm puts it, on "so-called youthful qualities, like quickness, adaptability, and physical vigor, which are the qualities needed in a world primarily orientated to success in competition rather than to the development of one's character."[5]

Silence may be interpreted either as an expression of quiet sympathy or of intense hate. By remaining silent, we may find that another will believe we are either in complete agreement with him or that every possibility of accord is excluded. It is generally assumed that silence is primal and that speaking emerged from silence. The Gospel of John tells us that in the "Beginning was the Word" but before that was the great silence, and Carlyle in *Our Heroes and Hero-Worship* says that speech is of time; silence is of eternity.

For psychological purposes we speak of different kinds and degrees of silence. Qualitatively silence may range from an appearance of coldness, sternness, defiance, disapproval or condemnation to calmness, warmth, approval, humility or excuse. In psychoanalysis, these different meanings and gradations of silence play important roles. As Reik has succinctly stated it, "In psychoanalysis, . . . what is spoken is not the most important thing. It appears to us more important to recognize what speech conceals and what silence reveals."[6]

Many people feel that psychoanalysis is mainly concerned with the *word* only. This is not necessarily true. The therapist, in relating to his patient as a human being, makes use not only of verbal interaction but of the many pauses, the subtle innuendoes, and especially the emotional effects of silence.

It may be said that the patient himself comes into therapy out of silence. His fears, anxieties and phobias are basically represented in the form of repressions and distortions of certain experiences, emotions and thoughts, most of which he has kept to himself. To his associates, he may seem a most garrulous person who talks a great deal about himself and his experiences; yet somehow his true inner feelings are submerged in his inner conscience where they remain silently repressed. It is only by a gradual unveiling of himself that he can talk in such a manner that his sounds begin to be perceptible in this zone of silence. In this context, the analyst listens not only to the *words* but also to *what the words do not say*. He listens with what Reik refers to as the "third ear," hearing not only what the patient says but also his inner voices as they emerge from his unconscious depths.

Listening to one's inner self is difficult because the voice often is distant, feeble and indistinct. The more removed we are from our real selves, the more we tend to retreat into our imaginations where the truth becomes camouflaged and deceptive to our ears. We listen only to what we feel we should be listening to, blocking and inhibiting many of those true messages and communications which seek to come from deep within us. Conversely, this process greatly interferes with the transmission of such utterances as are relayed to us from others and from the world about us. We find it difficult to be silent and to be aware of our innermost thoughts and beliefs. Instead we find the distorted and indirect expressions of our state of being verbalized in anxieties, bodily symptoms, vague and unspecified guilt feelings, and a general tiredness or restlessness. In short, conflicting thoughts and ideas of a strong and painful nature which should be felt consciously are silenced by superficial rationalizations and so find their expression in the form of fears, phobias and anxieties.

When conflicted, we are likely to deny life's problems by consciously silencing all discussion of them. Generally speaking, people shun talking about those problems which come close to the core of their beings. Try changing an ordinary conversation into something of a personal or intimate nature and see what happens. The moment the conversation becomes personal, the atmosphere grows tense and cautious. Such an intrusion is labeled poor tact and is considered an invasion of privacy. It is most definitely not the best way "to win friends and influence people."

Among primitive peoples and children, silence is deliberately used as a strategy to annihilate the opposition symbolically. Figuratively at least, as says Meerloo, "the enemy is 'cut dead.' Silence is an ostrich policy, a magical excommunication of angry ghosts. Don't talk about them—don't tempt fate by speaking of it . . . But the conspiracy of silence is still in our midst."[7] We all are aware of society's taboos on certain words and opinions. We just don't talk or write about them. We suppress and avoid them by the silence of conversation.

Silence, however, also has a specific healing and curative value in some particular situations. For instance, after a most painful emotional experience, verbal expression proves inadequate and so we feel forced to remain silent. The death of a loved one, the stress of an impending threat to our existence, intense hatred or shame or great feat— any one of these may bring about a protective need to withdraw completely and also dissolve the wish to communicate with others. However this wish to remain silent, to be alone and away from others, may be utilized constructively provided we do not exaggerate its true perspective and resort to self-pity and forced isolation.

H. G. Wells once said, "Words are sometimes only spoken to break the tension of silence, or to evade the conspiracy of silence." Unfortunately our fear of silence has become so intense that any pause, refusal to talk or to answer when we are expected to do so, is considered a betrayal and an excommunication of others. Feelings of intense nature such as affection or hostility are not verbalized at all. When in a state of doubt or confusion as to what reactions we might arouse in others, we hesitate before speaking and resort to silence and this, because of its painful effect on people, creates further tension and befuddlement, so setting into motion a vicious circle.

In stutterers, for instance, where self-expression is an agonizing ordeal, silence is most trying. Since the stutterer is so dependent upon words and has little self-evaluation of his own worth, silence threatens his need to know and hear what others might have to say about him. As long as he speaks, whether he stutters or not, he feels that his words act as a magic defense against danger or panic. To pause and remain silent leaves him open to the attack that he fears will come from without.

In more cultivated spheres of society, silence has always been more valued than speech. As the saying goes: speech is silver but silence is gold. The wise and scholarly man is he who is generally silent. Only after deep deliberation and after sizing up the situation squarely will he permit himself to speak, believing that "only a fool talks too soon and too much, since he cannot contain his knowledge," and that those who know the value of silence have acquired the secret of knowledge.

The Bible teaches us to be silent so that we may have an opportunity to listen with the ears of the soul. Silent reverence and meditation is of significant importance in many of our religious groups. A number of monastic orders require their members to maintain complete silence on the assumption that meaningless talk damages the soul. Since it is practically impossible for human beings to maintain a state of absolute non-communication, a complicated non-verbal gesture language has been developed in the place of oral conversation.

Still others feel that silence is deeper than speech and is the revelation of the creative unconscious. The Quakers, for instance, experience the initial moments of a silence as a unifying element. The act of prayer takes place when possible in an atmosphere of silence to protect us from disturbing noises and thoughts which might interfere with the necessary penetration into the depths of our being.

In Buddhism, the ultimate wisdom is Nirvana, which means the bringing of one's self to a minimum of desire and will. The less the will is excited, according to the Buddhists, the less one suffers. Through silence and meditation, so they believe, "the perfect calm of the spirit, deep rest, and inviolable confidence and serenity" are achieved.

Silence enables us to dissolve the barriers of our tensions and cautiousness, encouraging instead the integration and unification of our inner energies toward self-realization and inner communion. Silence also helps us toward self-awareness and to become more attentive and receptive to the truth. Emerson once said, "Happy is the hearing man; unhappy the speaking man. As long as I hear the truth, I am bathed by nature. The suggestions are thousandfold that I hear and see. The waters of the great deep have ingress and egress to the soul. But if I speak, I define, I confine, and am less."[8]

Through the constructive use of silence, we weave stronger ties with others and develop deeper feelings than words can possibly achieve. By silent contemplation too we are permitted to view others as they actually are, not as we wish they were. And as we relinquish whatever image of another we may have created in our illusions, we perceive in its place the genuine self of the person with whom we are trying to communicate.

179

Genuine understanding is facilitated only if we see one another realistically, each as a unique personality, apart from the subjective evaluation which past experience has helped us create. In order to foster such a state of mutual compatability, we should be content to be silent and listen with as few prejudices, condemnations and preconceived judgments as possible. Silence will then become an integrating and progressively unifying element in the ultimate growth of man.

I would like to conclude this chapter with the following description of silence as experienced by a patient of mine:—

> It is quiet, it is silent and the silence beats its own persistent tempo. It is a silence that mingles with aloneness but not loneliness. For to think, to feel, to sense, to love and to desire is to live often more fully than in a jungle of sound. There are no limits, no limitations— there is no void but space which is filled with a thousand tongues of wordless thought. It is a silence that cannot be created. It is sometimes come upon as a descending, invisible circle that encloses but does not bind—that surrounds but does not stifle. It is the imperceptible merging of the air with all infinity—the losing of one's identity but the becoming of one with all. The single cell of the being that becomes all cells of all things. It is a state that stops time and touches all of space. It is the heightening of the senses that is beyond reason and awareness. This kind of silence is rare, for the balance between being and non-being is so perfect that it cannot endure by the standards of known time-span. And so this irreducible perfection is the rarest of all gifts. To grasp it and be one with it is an experience never to be lost.

References

1. Peter Hobart Knapp: "The Ear, Listening and Hearing." *The Yearbook of Psychoanalysis*, Vol. X. New York, International Universities Press, Inc., 1954, p. 189.

2. Anne Morrow Lindbergh: *Gift from the Sea*. New York, Pantheon Books, Inc., 1955, p. 115.
3. George W. Crane: "Talk or Keep Quiet? Which?" Column, *Miami Herald*, August 1957.
4. Ved Mehta: *Face to Face*. Boston, Little Brown & Company, 1957, p. 142.
5. Erich Fromm: *Man for Himself*. New York, Rinehart and Company, 1947, p. 163.
6. Theodor Reik: *Listening with the Third Ear*. New York, Farrar, Straus, 1949, p. 126.
7. Joost A. M. Meerloo: *Conversation and Communication*. New Yord, International Universities Press, Inc., 1952, p. 115.
8. Ralph Waldo Emerson: *Essays*. Cuneo Press, Inc., 1936, p. 232.

When We Stop Listening

And if no one stops to listen, why of course a man will feel
All broke up and dislocated, and uneasy as an eel.
            —EUGENE FITCH WARE

W E stop listening and at once we cease to live realistically. We become afraid to listen to the truths about us, and in our frantic attempt to hold off fear and allay anxiety, we take refuge in rationalizations, blind spots, self denials and magic devices.

There are no magic or simple roads toward self-realization. That will come only through an exploration of the depths of the self—in the stripping away of the many obstructions hindering self-expression. To do this, we must learn to open our ears wide and to listen effectively to what goes on about us. Before we can achieve a real and complete awareness of *what is*, we must first look *actively* within ourselves and there seek for the constructive truth about ourselves and the world we live in.

As long as we are compelled to seek beyond ourselves, we will continue to avoid coming to grips with our true selves and we shall bottle up whatever creative energies we have available for productive living. If we would overcome these handicaps, it is essential that we turn away from the periphery of our personalities, and live more healthily at the center of our beings. Only then shall we listen with our *hearts* rather than with our *heads*.

In our blind quest for complete and personal tranquility, we have only added greater confusion to our lives. In the struggle for the ultimate in truth and happiness, we

182

have lost many of our true feelings and values and so find ourselves increasingly involved in confusions, uncertainties and frustrations. In the denial of our everyday struggles and inner conflicts, we have become as so many spectator-like automatons, characterized by passivity, futility, shallow living and emptiness.

It is difficult for most of us to accept pain and suffering as integral parts of living. Instead we search frantically for new ways of achieving a so-called *peace of mind*. To find this, we turn to religion, "how-to" books, sex, alcohol, and even—in the past three or four years—to tranquilizers. In an article published in *Fortune* (May 1957), Francis Bello estimated that some 20,000,000 Americans have used tranquilizers, while the sales for the same year totalled about $175,000,000. And Max Lerner, in a stimulating article in the *New York Post* entitled "Packaged Peace of Mind," wrote: "The drug firms have fallen upon a bonanza, and they are working it for all its worth, in an advertising-and-promotion campaign for such brand names as Thorazine, Equinal, Atarax, Serpasil, and Miltown, promising relief for everything from infantile colic to senile anxiety and for most emotional complaints in between the two."[1]

The danger involved here is that these tranquilizers *fail* to get at the core of the difficulty, and whatever temporary peace of mind they bring is but a "packaged" peace of mind. The road to true happiness cannot be bought at ten cents for a pill! A "happy" pill is only a makeshift solution, never a lasting one. As Lerner went on to point out: "This is the road to packaged conformity. Those who are today lulled into a sense of tranquility through buying something they will swallow and produce changes in their central and autonomic nervous systems may tomorrow buy and swallow a packaged social nostrum. In both cases they will feel that it is unnecessary to strive and fight to slap the dragons by will and courage. It

183

will no longer interest them much, for all dragons will seem unreal, and the only reality will be packaged tranquility as advertised."[2]

As long as we resort to such false manipulators of the mind as tranquilizers, we shall never listen or perceive effectively. In the severing of the central from the autonomic nervous system, we disturb the normal connections of adaptation between the forepart and the primitive back section of the human brain. This forepart which contains the mechanisms of human choice, selective listening, will and social intelligence, is—as Bello maintains—the part on which mankind has relied for the first million years and will have to rely for the next million.

In our present day culture, we are so accustomed to listening to the sounds and voices of those around us that, in ignoring the echoes of our own inner perceptions, we tend to become deafened to them and to move away from our true innermost feelings and beliefs. The furtheraway we move, the more dependent we become on the voices of others. We create, as a result, a state of loneliness and forced isolation, for once we learn to lean on others, we find it difficult to come back to ourselves.

Most of us fear moving away from such stock opinions, customs, or beliefs as we have come to accept as gospel truths. Confronted with new ideas or changing experiences, we easily become strained and conflicted, and we fear and, for the most part, avoid seeing or listening to anything which might interfere with our preconceived notions. We remain fixed in the past, afraid to live in the present, and so we become inwardly tense, afraid, confused and frustrated. Experiencing anything new as a threat, we develop suspicious attitudes toward whatever seems to us to be an invasion. New truths can be accepted only if we have the courage and the flexibility to adapt ourselves to the constant changes about us and can make ourselves aware of reality as an ever-moving dynamic

184

process. If we instead become dogmatic and prejudiced, we close our minds and our ears against the outside world and ultimately *cease to listen.*

In listening effectively, spontaneous action is always the best. To perceive fully and communicate productively with others, it is essential that we make available to ourselves the full potential of our creative energies, that we force ourselves to be as open-minded as possible, and that we avoid too quick criticism and fixed judgments. Rather than remaining passive, detached or resigned to the world and its influx of messages, we must develop that sense of alive eagerness, curiosity and vigilance which will give zest to our intellects and continually accelerate our listening operation.

Today we are becoming helpless victims of a mechanistic society. We evaluate ourselves mainly in terms of materialistic values, measuring satisfaction as a means to an end rather than as a relatedness and feeling for one's self. We act like machines, rarely experiencing ourselves as *we are.* Instead we see ourselves as we *think* we are supposed to be. In this milieu of false values, we have moved away from the center of our beings, resorting to more superficial and externalized living. Meaningless chatter has replaced communicative speech, and too little effective listening or inner reflection is taking place. As a result of this progressive deterioration of our true selves, we are simultaneously suffering an impairment of spontaneity and a loss of individuality which are gradually leading to a moral and humanistic breakdown.

In our fears and inability to remain alone with ourselves long enough to listen to the voice of our inner conscience, we are slowly crippling those forces which should be made available for productive living, happiness and psychic health. In achieving these, mere superficial insight or conscious awareness is not enough. To be effective, insight must contain elements that are sensitive and mature;

it must spring from within the innermost self; and, most important, it must be associated with a desire to engage in a vital struggle to gain health and happiness, rather than on any "packaged peace-of-mind."

The decision as to the level of active existence we shall find the most productive and capable of providing the highest degree of satisfaction, is something each of us must make for himself. Self-realization cannot be measured in terms of social or universal values. The individual must *want* to discipline himself to listen to himself and to put a real value on his life and happiness; he must have the courage to face himself as *he is* and not as he feels he *should be*. Whatever results will be dependent upon his will to listen earnestly to himself, to face inner truths, to relinquish his illusions about himself and, ultimately, to *be* himself.

We live today in a technological world where we worship gadgets—jet planes which break through sound barriers; long sleek automobiles that are difficult to park; television sets that can be operated electronically from contour chairs. In this age of speed and action, we find that we have too *little time to stop to listen to ourselves* or to take time for quiet thought. Instead of seeing ourselves as independent identities with thoughts, beliefs and feelings of our own, we seek constantly for prestige, social standing and success, a situation which blocks any real evaluation or feeling for self identification. In our struggle for social survival, we become alienated and wholly dependent upon others, seeing ourselves as we think others see us. In this process of externalized living, we tend to neglect our true selves and we become further alienated, estranged, and distant from others.

The more empty we become as individuals, the less we tend to listen with selective purpose. We seem to be more interested in achieving comfort and being passively entertained, than in any real effort toward concentration.

186

Attempts are made by society, at every instance, to give us commodities to *attract* the attention without actually *engaging* it, to entertain rather than give us the means to *involve* ourselves actively or create a desire to *challenge*. In our urgency to grasp everything within our reach, we emphasize increasingly the sense of our own "efficiency" by subordinating ourselves to the errorless perfection of a machine. Heedless of the truths within ourselves, we place books and distractions in the path of our listening, and so widen the gap between our true and our idealized selves.

Basically lazy, we also cease to listen when things which we do not understand become complex or require some extra concentrated effort on our part. With neither the time nor the patience to listen, those messages which disturb our fixed and preconceived notions or ideas, are rejected almost as if we had deliberately plugged our ears. Furthermore, we allow our minds to be filled with resentments, blind justifications and conflicting attitudes which disturb effective listening and lead toward confusion, misunderstandings and further tensions.

How many of us as parents wrongly evaluate our own children and judge them mistakenly because we assess their actions in terms of our own past prejudices rather than in relation to the true actualities. A New York subway poster for the prevention of juvenile delinquency makes this point in the query: "Are You Too Old to Listen to Kid's Stuff?" As long as we continue to listen to our children from adult levels and refuse to recognize the fact that where listening should be effective as a give-and-take exchange, juvenile problems will continue to exist.

Many problems in bringing up our children will be simplified when we learn how to listen and how to use our listening abilities constructively. There is no doubt that as individuals, we hear only what we want to hear, and discard whatever we may feel to be disturbing or harmful to our ears. Many parents will argue that they listen all day long. True, we are ever-present sounding boards. But how often do we listen effectively to the deep-down problems that may be disturbing our children[4] Let us try to figure out why, and how we can create better listening atmospheres with our children.

First of all, we must find time in our busy day to be alone with them. During this period we must make every effort to remove outside noises and distractions of the radio, television, the barking of the dog, the sound of the kitchen fan and so on, so as to create a quieting, comforting and relaxing effect. Finally, there must exist, between parent and child, a feeling of mutual respect, intimacy, freedom of expression, and a deep sense of relatedness. Once this feeling of togetherness and natural contact has been established, the listening exchange will be at its highest working capacity and positive communion and communication achieved. From here on in, both parent and child will develop a sense of sympathy, confidence and understanding, one for the other.

Considerable attention is being focused today on family communication and its positive aspects on family life. One specialist has suggested that both amusement and considerable enlightenment may be had in taping a number of spontaneous family discussions and then playing them back, and all concerned listening insofar as possible with open minds and ears to hear themselves just as others hear them.

An analysis of two hundred such tape recordings of family table talk, made by Dr. James H. S. Bossard of the University of Pennsylvania and reported earlier this year in *Presbyterian Life*, revealed certain definite patterns of talking and listening. There were some families who exchanged little more than short, sharp "yes's," "no's," "wh-huh's" and "please pass the salt." Others utilized

188

their time airing current family grievances and reliving past ones. Another segment was equally critical but released its attacks outward. Here the family habit of disparagement, the attitude of belittlement, was no different from the second group's except that its victims were the neighbors, the teachers, community leaders and so on. In the recordings there were also bits of news, jokes, pleasantries and reports of successes. Honest and thoughtful reactions to public issues were discussed; as well as disagreements and problems. There was a marked difference here which was in both quality and the tone in which they were offered and responded to.

As Dr. Bossard pointed out, it would seem that most families habitually talk in the same way, and almost without exception about the same things. However, since the family group is probably not aware of these habits, of what they indicate about basic family attitudes or of what they can do to the life of the family and the development of its members, listening with this "third ear" to *what is said*—and *how*—within the home give its adult members one more gauge for evaluating the all-over pattern of family life and how constructively they are going about achieving their ends.

The importance of good listening as an effective tool in learning is becoming more acceptable and recognizable today than ever before. Present day systems of aural communication—radio, television, sound movies—have only been made available to ourselves and our children within the last few decades. The recent study, "Mass Communication and Education," released by the Educational Policies Commission, revealed that the average public school student now spends from two to four hours a day listening to and watching TV. As a result, the children of today have ever-broadening horizons and an increasing awareness about present-day world and local situations.

189

According to one British communications expert, we are able to absorb and store away in our brains some *ten billion pieces* of information, one piece for each of the brain's nerve cells. But, it is inconceivable that anyone—even the greatest genius—has that much information tucked away in his brain. However, that this amazing feat is possible—if not probable—is primarily due to two factors—availability and mental receptivity. For instance, reading is about the fastest method for acquiring information. If we were to read and take in twenty-five pieces of information each second, it would take eight hours of such intake each day for forty years to fill the brain. But, according to Dr. I. J. Good, of the Government Communication Headquarters, even if we could take in the maximum amount of information, we might still be uninformed. For the crux of memory is the ability to tap the cells of stored information and to so activate them that their contents can be made available when we want them.

Much more receptive to taking in information than it is to giving it up, the brain may be compared to a two-way highway—the entering lane clear and straight, while the returning lane is devious and filled with obstacles. This being so, when we are faced with an apparent loss of memory, we would do well to seek another route away from the storage cell. This is just another way of describing what happens when we listen with purpose or when we are selective.

Once this phase of constructive listening has become fixed, our conscious thinking is able to move in and assimilate the information we take in by generalizing, by abstracting, by looking for fundamentals. In this fashion, the thinking process actually reduces the amount of information we have selected for use or for storing away in our brains. And in this same context, the fewer lapses and distractions we have present when listening and concentrating, the more interest and incentive there is in remembering.

The perfection and the use of the intellect alone, however, inhibits deep communication. In order to attempt more effective communicating, there must also be present the process of feeling *with* and *in* things. A genuine basis for understanding and communication will then be possible. Once this has been experienced, according to Meerloo, "the way to the world lies open. Understanding is pausing momentarily, stepping outside the continual stream of occurrences to observe the passing stream. He who always runs through life never learns to understand anyone else."[3]

The more we attempt to understand each other, the better we can communicate. Good understanding means freeing oneself of words as such, and the strengthening of our capacities for real listening and an intuitive feeling and respect for others.

To discover order and honesty in his perceiving, Man must have the courage to face the truth within himself. His listening must remain free of prejudiced distortions, false condemnations, and personal resentments. Furthermore, he must be honest enough to develop a realistic understanding of his own motives and the actions to which he is driven by them. The more able he is to listen on a rational, responsible and humanistic basis, the more readily will Man ultimately realize himself and discover his most constructive possibilities.

The more we tend toward health and self-realization, the better listeners we will become, the more we will live in the present and the less we will communicate in terms of the past. And the more relaxed, spontaneous, alive and productive we become, the more effective will we be able to listen and the better able will we be to tap further our hidden sources of creative energies. We can then give of ourselves more freely in conversation, retreat

191

less often behind empty word systems, and so develop a sense of mutual understanding and rapport. In order that this may become a reality, we must practice the art of listening. Only then shall we face the truth within ourselves, and avoid self-betrayal through falsities, illusions, rationalizations and neurotic solutions.

References

1, 2. Max Lerner: "Packaged Peace of Mind." *New York Post*, June 25, 1957.
3. J. A. M. Meerloo: *Conversation and Communication*. New York, International Universities Press, Inc., 1956, p. 194.

Bibliography

ADLER, ALFRED: *The Practice and Theory of Individual Psychology.* Tr. by P. Rodin. New York, Harcourt, Brace, 1924.

ANGYAL, A.: *Foundations for a Science of Personality.* New York, The Commonwealth Fund, New York, 1941.

BARBARA, DOMINICK A.: *Stuttering: A Psychodynamic Approach to Its Understanding and Treatment.* New York, Julian Press, 1954.

...............: *Your Speech Reveals Your Personality.* Springfield, Illinois, Charles C Thomas, Publisher, 1958.

BENEDICT, RUTH F.: *Patterns of Culture.* Boston, Houghton Mifflin, 1934.

BRAATY, TRYGVE: *Fundamentals of Psychoanalytic Technique.* New York, John Wiley & Sons, Inc., 1954.

BYNNER, WITTER: *The Way of Life according to Laotzu.* New York, The John Day Company, 1944.

CANNON, W. B.: *Bodily Changes in Pain, Hunger, Fear and Rage.* New York, Appleton, 1929.

...............: *The Wisdom of the Body.* New York, Norton, 1932.

CHASE, STUART: *The Tyranny of Words.* New York, Harcourt, Brace, 1938.

CHISHOLM, FRANCIS P.: *Introductory Lectures on General Semantics.* Chicago, Institute of General Semantics, 1944.

COBB, STANLEY: *Borderlines of Psychiatry.* Cambridge, Mass., Harvard University Press, 1944.

DUNBAR, FLANDERS: *Emotions and Bodily Changes. A Survey of Literature on Psychosomatic Interrelationships.* 1910-1945. 3rd ed. New York, Columbia University Press, 1946.

FADIMAN, CLIFTON: *Party of One.* New York, World Publishing Company, 1955.

FENICHEL, OTTO: *The Psychoanalytic Theory of Neurosis.* New York, W. W. Norton & Company, Inc., 1945.

FREUD, SIGMUND: *A General Introduction to Psychoanalysis.* New York, Liveright, 1935.

FROMM, ERICH: *The Forgotten Language.* New York, Rinehart & Company, 1951.

.................: *Man for Himself.* New York, Rinehart & Company, 1947.

.................: *The Art of Loving.* New York, Harper & Bros., 1958.

GESELL, ARNOLD and ILG, FRANCES L.: *The Child from Five to Ten.* New York, Harper & Bros., 1946.

GOLDSTEIN, KURT: *The Organism.* New York, American Book Company, 1939.

HAYAKAWA, S. I.: *Language in Action.* New York, Harcourt, Brace & Company, Inc., 1943.

HORNEY, KAREN: *Neurosis and Human Growth.* New York, W. W. Norton & Company, Inc., 1950.

.................: *The Neurotic Personality of Our Time.* New W. Norton & Company, Inc., 1938.

.................: *Our Inner Conflicts.* New York, W. W. Norton & Company, Inc., 1945.

HUXLEY, A.: *The Art of Seeing.* New York, Harper & Bros., 1942.

JASTROW, JOSEPH: *Effective Thinking.* New York, World Publishing Company, 1931.

JOHNSTON, WENDELL: *People in Quandaries.* New York, Harper & Bros., 1948.

.................: *Your Most Enchanted Listener.* New York, Harper & Bros., 1956.

KANNER, LEO: *Child Psychiatry.* Springfield, Illinois, Charles C Thomas, 1942.

KASANNIN, J. S.: *Language and Thought in Schizophrenia.* Collected Papers. California, University of California Press, 1944.

KORZYBSKI, ALFRED: *Science and Sanity: An Introduction to Non-Aristotelian Systems and General Semantics.* Lancaster, Science Press, 2nd ed., 1941

KRISHNAMURTI, J.: *The First and Last Freedom.* New York, Harper & Bros., 1954.

LEE, IRVING J.: *Language Habits in Human Affairs.* New York, Harper & Bros., 1951.

LINDBERGH, ANNE MORROW: *Gift from the Sea.* New York, Pantheon Books, 1955.

MACMURRAY, JOHN: *Reason and Emotion.* New York, D. Appleton-Century, 1938.

MALINOWSKI, BRONISLAW: *Magic, Science and Religion.* New York, Doubleday Anchor Books, 1954.

MEERLOO, J. A. M.: *Conversation and Communication — A Psychological Inquiry into Language and Human Relations.* New York, International Universities Press, 1952.

MURROW, EDWARD R.: *This I Believe.* New York, Simon and Schuster, 1952.

NICHOLS, RALPH G. and STEVENS, LEONARD A.: *Are You Listening?* New York, McGraw-Hill Book Company, Inc., 1957.

OLIVER, ROBERT T.: *The Psychology of Persuasive Speech.* New York, Longmans, Green & Company, 2nd ed., 1957.

PIAGET, JEAN: *The Language and Thought of the Child.* New York, Harcourt, Brace & Company, 1926.

REIK, THEODOR: *Listening with the Third Ear.* New York, Farrar, Straus and Company 1949

RIESMAN, DAVID *et al.: The Lonely Crowd.* New York, Doubleday & Company, Inc., 1955

ROGERS, CARL R.: *Counseling and Psychotherapy.* Boston, Houghton Mifflin, 1942.

RUESCH, JURGEN, and BATESON, GREGORY: *Communication: The Social Matrix of Psychiatry.* New York, Norton & Company, 1951.

...............: *Disturbed Communication.* New York, Norton & Company, 1957

TRAVIS, LEE EDWARD: Editor—*Handbook of Speech Pathology.* New York, Appleton-Century-Crofts, Inc., 1957.

VON BERTALANFFY, L.: *Problems of Life.* New York, John Wiley and Sons, Inc., 1932.

WELLS, H. G., HUXLEY, J. S., and WELLS, G. P.: *The Science of Life.* New York, The Literary Guild, 1934.

WHITEHEAD, ALFRED NORTH: *Science and the Modern World.* New York, The Macmillan Company, 1925.

WHYTE, L. L.: *The Unitary Principle in Physics and Biology.* New York, Henry Holt & Company, 1949.

195

WIENER, N.: *The Human Use of Human Beings—Cybernetics and Society*. Boston, Houghton Mifflin, 1950.

WOLBERG, L. R.: *Technique of Psychotherapy*. New York, Grune & Stratton, 1954.

ZILBOORG, G.: *A History of Medical Psychology*. New York, Norton & Company, 1941.

Index

A

Abstractions, 35
Acknowledgment, 83-85, 145
Adler, A., 193
Angyal, A., 193
Aristotle, 53
Art, practice of, 1
Attention, 3
  listening and, 88
Auditory
  hallucinations, 30
  repression, 166
Authority, 53-54

B

Barbara, D. A., 1-3
Barnett, R., 47
Bateson, G., 195
Bell, A. G., 22
Bello, F., 183, 184
Benchley, R., 126
Benedict, R. F., 193
von Bertalanffy, L., 195
"Blab," 171
Block, M., 96
Bores, 56
Bossard, J. H. S., 188, 189
Braaty, T., 193
Brain, 90, 91, 184, 190
Briffault, 79
Bynner, W., 193

C

Cannon, W. B., 193
Cardano of Padua, 22

Carlyle, 175
Chase, S., 193
Chatterboxes, 126
Chesterton, G. K., 149
Child
  listening and, 101-105
  magic and, 71-74
Chisholm, F. P., 193
Cicero, 53, 149
Cobb, S., 193
Cochlea, 19-20
Communication
  aim of, 10
  animals and, 16
  complacency in, 119
  disagreement in, 7
  efficiency of, 8
  effective, 6-9, 58
  evaluation in, 7-8
  family, 102, 188-189
  mutual, 11
  negative approach to, 147
  psychotherapy and, 151-165
  resigned person and, 140
  with self, 32, 33, 34
  social, 169, 171
  successful, 8, 82
Compliancy, 119-120
Comprehension, 3-4, 148
  definition of, 5
"Compulsive nodders," 113, 114
Concentration, 2-3, 141, 149, 187
  lack of, 2
Conflicts, listener and, 134
Consciousness, stream of, 91-93
Crane, G. W., 169, 181
Cybernetics, 39

D

Dalgaino, 22
Deaf
  children, 26
  "depression of," 25
  "ear," listening with, 138-150
  education of, 21-22
Deafness
  hysterical, 25, 111
  psuedo, 138
Dependent listener, 116-118
Discipline, 1
Disraeli, 32
Distractions, 108, 115, 142
  listening and, 2
Dostoyevsky, 11
Dreams, sound and, 167
Dunbar, F., 193

E

Ear
  attuned, listening with, 46-48
  human, 17-21
    inner, 17-18, 19
      fluid of, 19
      listening with, 32-48
    middle, 17, 18
    outer, 17
      listening with, 14-31
    symbolic meaning of, 14, 15
  trumpet, 18
Eardrum, 17, 18, 19
Earring, 15-16
Emerson, R. W., 65, 179, 181
Emotions
  disturbed, 135
  persuasive speech and, 63
Euphemism, 76
Eustachian tube, 18

F

Fadiman, C., 115, 125, 1-3
Falstaff, 97
Fears, 24

F

Feedback
  mcehanism, 8, 39-41
  defective, 140,147
  external, 40
  internal, 40
  selective, 41
Fenestra
  ovalis, 18, 19
  rotunda, 19
Fenichel, O., 193
Ferenczi, 71
"Filling sounds," 16
Free-associations, 155
Freud, S., 28, 29, 107, 153, 194
Fromm, E., 1, 13, 175, 181, 194
Frustration, 108-109

G

Gallaudet, E. M., 22
Gesell, A., 24, 31, 72, 194
Goldstein, K., 194
Good, I. J., 190
Graham, B., 49

H

Hayakawa, S. I., 64, 1-4
Hearing, 14
  development of, 22-23
  impairment of, 21-22
  psychological
    aspects of, 22-30
    levels of, 23
Heinicke, 22
Henry, M., 138
Henry, R., 6, 10, 13
Hitler, 55
Hogeman, S. M., 166
Home, art of listening in, 101-102
Horney, K., 12, 13, 42, 147, 150, 194
Hostility, 122-123
Hughes, C. E., 1 9
Humility, listening with, 3
Huxley, A., 54, 194
Huxley, J. S., 30, 195

198

I

Ilg, F., *24*, *31*, *72*, *1–4*
Incus, 19
Individual, listener as, 10-13
Inferences, 61-62
Inner vitality, 6
Integrity of others, 11
Intelligence, listening and, 93
Interests, 6
Interpersonal network, 151
"Interpretative cortex," 92
Intrapersonal network, 151
Introspection, 147
Isakower, O., 28, 30, 107

J

Janet, P. F., *69*
Jastrow, J., 74, 79, 194
Johnson, L., 56
Johnson, W., 5, 13, 40, 48, 49, 53, 64, 151
Johnston, W., 194
Jones, E., 14

K

Kanner, L., *30*, *1–4*
Kasannin, J. S., 194
Knapp, P. H., 26, 30, 166, 167, 180
Korzybski, A., 194
Krishnamurti, J., ii, 194
Kubwonebu, 70

L

de L'Epee, *22*
Langer, S., 36
Language, 9, 145, 154
Laurence, W. L., 91, 96
Learning, listening in, 189
Lee, I., 109, 112, 194
Lerner, M., 183, 192
Levy-Bruhl, 67
Lindbergh, A. M., 168, 181, 195

Listener
  compulsive, 50
  good, 4
  as individual, 10-13
  ineffectual, 3
  partial, 140
  poor, 4, 43-46, 128, 131
    emotional or over-anxious type, 45-46
    intellectual or logical type, 44
  productive, 3
Listening
  art of, 1-13
  attentive, 88
  curative value of, 95-96
  with deaf ear, 138-150
  distractive, 46
  effectively, 80, 81, 133, 185
    blockages to, 108-112
  to essence of things, 80-96
  faulty, origins of, 100
  fully, 80
  good, communicative aspects of, 6-13
  holistic, 80, 105
  improving skill of, 93-95
  with inner ear, 32-48
  magic of, 85-79
  with modest ear, 113-125
  nonparticipation, 140-141
  non-verbal, 59-63
  not, 182-192
    disease of, 97-112
  to oneself, 174
  with outer ear, 14-31
  productive, 11
    essentials of, 1-6, 12-13
  with rebellious ear, 126-137
  with receptive ear, 49-64
  resigned, 138
  selective, 86-91
  serious, 2
  skill in, 1
  with "static," 41-46
  subjective, 42
  superficial, 2
  with third ear, 151-165

199

vicarious, 80
"Logos," doctrine of, 65
Lytton, E. B., 4

M

Macmurray, J., 1–5
Magic
  child's use of, 71-74
  language of, 66
  primitive, 67-68
Malinowski, B., 66, 67, 79, 195
Malleus, 19
Mann, T., 52
Mark, 14, 80
Meaning, shared, 9
Meditation, 173
Mediums, 69
Merloo, J. A. M., 14, 17, 30, 55, 58,
    4, 73, 79, 158, 165, 177,
    181, 191, 192, 195
Midas, 15
Mind, listening and, 6
Moro reflex, 22
Motion conception, hearing and, 29
Murrow, E. R., 4, 195

N

Need to be heard, 56–59
Nichols, R. G., 4, 13, 90, 93, 96,
    97, 99, 112, 195

O

Objectivity, 5
Oliver, R. T., 52, 64, 88, 96, 111,
    112, 195
Otosclerosis, 21

P

Paget, R., 60
Parent-child lisenting relationship,
    87, 102-104, 187-188
Participation, active, in listening, 3,
    143

Patience, 2
Peace of mind, 183, 186
Penfield, W., 91, 92
Perception, 62, 88-89, 151
Persuasion, 51-56
Piaget, J., 195
Pigors, 54
Plutarch, 113
Propaganda, 54, 55
Psychic health, 27, 38
Psychoanalysis, silence in, 175
Psychotherapy, 151
  listening in, 153

R

Radio, listening ability and, 105–106
Ramsdell, D. A., 25, 30
Rankin, P. T., 98
Reading, speed in, 90
Rebellious individual, 126-137
Reflection, 2, 185
Reik, T., 165, 175, 176, 181, 195
Resigned person, 138-150
Riesman, D., 195
Road toward inner freedom, 162-165
Rogers, C. R., 195
Reusch, J., 22, 44, 48, 82, 83, 85,
    96, 108, 112, 125, 145, 150,
    195

S

Schilder, 166
Scott, W., 1
Seeing, 14
Self-effacing individual, 117-125
Self-evaluation, 6
Self-expression, 155, 173
Self-knowledge, 12
Self-realization, 164, 182-183, 186,
    191
Sensory receptors in communication,
    141
Shakespeare, 56
Silence
  art of, 167

200

constructive use of, 179
creative, 170
curative value of, 177
fear of, 174, 178
kinds of, 175
productive, 168
in religion, 178, 179
sound of, 166-181
Silent
  observer, 155
  retreat, 170
Silverman, S. R., 21, 30
Sleep, sound and, 166, 167
Socrates, 49, 60
Sound
  of silence, 166-181
  waves, 1, 19
Sounds, fear of, 24
Speakers, influential, 113-114
Speech, 33, 36
  faculty of, 71-72
  persuasive, 5-56
  rate of, 4, 90
Stapes, 18
Static, 123, 146
Stevens, L. A., 4, 12, 90, 93, 96, 97,
    99, 112, 195
Stutterers, silence and, 178
Superstition, logic of, 74-76
Symbolizing, 36
Symbols, 34, 35, 36, 37

T

Taft, C. P., 63
Talk, 168-169
Tangenital
  reply, 85
  response, 87
Teen-agers, listening and, 99-100
Telekinesis, 68, 69
Therapeutic process, listening in,
    154-156
Therapist
  anxious, over-talkative, 160

as a listener, 157
"so-called" silent, 161-162
soothing, 162
Therapy, disturbed listening posts in,
    158-162
Thinking, rate of, 4
"Third ear," 151-165
Tranquilizers, 183-184
Travis, L. E., 34, 38, 195
Trobriand Islands, 67, 69-71

U

Understanding, 11, 180, 1-1

V

Van Horne, H., 51, 64
Ved Mehta, 170, 181
Verbocracy, 55
Verbosity, 55
Von Frisch, 16

W

Wallace, M., 126
Wallenberg, M., 28, 31
Ware, E. F., 182
W ssel, B., 159, 165
Welles, O., 80
Wells, G. P., 30, 195
Wells, H. G., 30, 50, 177, 195
Whitehead, A. N., 195
Whyte, L. L., 195
Wiener, N., 39, 196
Wolberg, L. R., 196
Words
  meaning of, 6-7
  power of, 65
  social taboos on, 76-79

Z

Zilboorg, G., 196